Praise for
Practical Mindfulness

"Dr. Sazima brings mindfulness down to its nuts and bolts and out of the lofty air where it too often floats out of reach. He speaks from the heart, not just as a physician, but as a patient who found benefit through meditative practice and brought those techniques to patients with medical and mental disorders. At times solemn, at times irreverent, but always genuine, he's put it all here on the page. Read it, but more importantly, do it."

—**Chris Aiken, MD**, psychiatrist, director of the Mood Treatment Center, Wake Forest University School of Medicine; editor-in-chief, Carlat Psychiatry Report; author, *Bipolar, Not So Much: Understanding Your Mood Swings and Depression*

"*Practical Mindfulness* is a clearly written guide to the practice of meditation and mindfulness. Step by step, Dr. Sazima leads us through exercises that lead to deeper meditation, while at the same time describing the philosophy behind mindfulness drawing on a wide range of concepts from quantum physics to neuroanatomy. The book is written in clear language with a dollop of humor so that it succeeds in being not only informative, but also entertaining. Anyone who reads *Practical Mindfulness* will find it an indispensable guide to leading a more mindful life."

—**John O'Neal, MD,** psychiatrist, Sacramento, CA; coauthor of *Handbook of Clinical Psychopharmacology for Therapists*

"As a psychiatrist, I regularly recommend mindfulness meditation because I know I am supposed to, but I always felt intimidated when I would try it myself. Dr. Sazima's humor and humanity make this practical guide just the right place to start, or jumpstart, your own mindfulness practice. *Practical Mindfulness* is the one book I recommend to my patients, even when they don't believe they want to start meditating."

—**Lisa Goldstein, MD,** child and adolescent psychiatrist, Philadelphia, PA

"I wholeheartedly recommend Dr. Greg Sazima's book, *Practical Mindfulness*. It is an extremely user-friendly book that is essential to both everyday users who need new skills for how to be 'in the here and now' and deal with stress, as well as a wonderful read for mental health professionals to add to their tool bag of counseling skills. I teach Motivational Psychology and plan to add this book as required reading for both my undergraduate and graduate students."

—**Holly Davani, MA, HPI,** certified behavioral trainer, Baltimore, MD; associate graduate faculty, Department of Psychology, Towson University

"What a delightful, fun and informative book. It's a very practical guide for anyone wanting to learn more about meditation and for anyone wanting to enhance their experience with meditation. Dr. Sazima has a great way with words and takes you on an enjoyable journey to enlightenment, peace, and harmony. As someone who meditates daily, I thoroughly enjoyed the book and will recommend it to all my friends, family, colleagues, and clients."

—**Roland Williams, MA, LAADC, NCACII, CADCII, ACRPS, SAP,** master addictions counselor, educator, consultant; author of *Recovery is a Verb*

"*Practical Mindfulness* is a gem of a book designed to help physicians incorporate mindfulness into their practices and lives. Greg Sazima knows his audience. He writes with wisdom, insight, and humor and in an original voice. This practical and highly readable book integrates helpful case examples and exercises with mindfulness knowledge."

—**Melanie Greenberg, PhD,** psychotherapist, Marin, CA;
author, *The Stress-Proof Brain*

"All voices are needed to share the practices of mindfulness and meditation widely. Based on years of mindfulness practice from his own life and teaching others, Dr Sazima shares mindfulness in his 'no-nonsense, no-incense' unique voice. *Practical Mindfulness* can be the portal to mindfulness for those who are still looking for a different kind of voice to invite them in."

—**Lenna L. Liu, MD, MPH,** pediatrician, Seattle, WA;
professor of pediatrics, University of Washington School
of Medicine

"Dr. Sazima has taken on a potentially intimidating, complex concept and has created a practical, approachable guide to meditation and mindfulness. After reading *Practical Mindfulness*, I feel more confident that I can incorporate this practice in my own life, and I will share these techniques with my patients as well."

—**George P. Kent, MD,** family physician, San Jose, CA;
teaching faculty, Stanford/O'Connor Family Medicine
Residency Program

"Surgical patients must deal with physical and psychological pain before and after surgery. The ability to manage these real challenges with meditation rather than medication can be very beneficial to the surgical patient. Dr. Sazima, through lifelong learning and personal experience provides in *Practical Mindfulness* a practical guide on therapeutic meditation that will be useful to my patients."

—**Rick Nedelman, MD, FACS,** general surgeon, Springfield, OH; assistant clinical professor of surgery, Wright State University

"Dr. Sazima's witty, clear-eyed guide to mindfulness is all the novice needs to dive in, with a logical framework and a writing style that brings a smile to nearly every page. Sure, it's practical, but also insightful and entertaining. It's the mindfulness guide I've been waiting to be available for my patients, and even physician colleagues that want to learn more. No more excuses, now that *Practical Mindfulness* is there for us!"

—**Eric Mankin, MD,** family physician; president, Main Line Health Care, Philadelphia, MA

"*Practical Mindfulness* is an example of 'teaching a person to fish.' By communicating with clarity and humor, Dr. Sazima provides tangible skills that can improve life for busy and often stressed clinicians— and our patients. Armed with strategies, medical providers can help patients and families use mindful practices in managing disease and promoting wellness. *Practical Mindfulness* will help the open-minded clinician pay it forward."

—**Christopher F. Bolling, MD, FAAP**, pediatrician, Crestview Hills, KY; professor of pediatrics, University of Cincinnati College of Medicine

"*Practical Mindfulness* is a resource for those of us who thought meditation was for 'other people.' Thankfully, Dr. Sazima makes the point strongly that anyone can learn to meditate and ultimately benefit from it. The information is clearly presented and refreshingly without religious or New Age overtones. This is both a 'how to' guide as well as a very digestible discussion of how meditation works from the neuropsychiatric standpoint. Our patients who suffer chronic pain and anxiety may particularly benefit, but this is also a nice guide for all of us."

—**Paul Vargo, MD**, gastroenterologist, Saint Paul, MN

"*Practical Mindfulness* is a book like no other...it is not simply a manual, and it is not just a garden-variety cookbook—yet it affords the reader a pragmatic approach to meditation and health benefits in a unique way. It is part history, part philosophy, part popular culture, part science—all presented in a witty and informative style. There are multiple layers, and one must carefully digest its contents, lest the reader miss important nuances and provocative concepts."

—**Jong Rho, MD**, pediatric neurologist, San Diego, CA; Professor, UC San Diego School of Medicine

"*Practical Mindfulness* is likely to become a treasure for many. Dr. Greg Sazima infuses his extensive training and knowledge of the mind and body and creates a 'no-nonsense' guide to help others get their minds and bodies right. What's unique about Sazima's approach is not just his abiding insistence that meditation unlocks the key to happiness, tranquility, centeredness, even gratitude. Others have done this to be sure, but Sazima's humor, much of it directed himself and his training, adds an air of authenticity and a sense that he, like the rest of us, is just trying to figure it out. That said, this is not just a book but a tool for figuring things out."

—**Steve Barrett**, educator, Columbus, OH; superintendent, Gahanna-Jefferson Public Schools

"In *Practical Mindfulness*, Dr. Greg Sazima explores the strategies that can lead students—and teaching professionals—to a broader and more graceful understanding of where we fit in an ever-changing and complex world. Dr. Saz does so with compassion, humor and a little welcome snark. Mindfulness is the practice of stepping off the treadmill of study or career and seeking a grounding in the home that is the inner self. It is something not easily or shallowly assessed, but the important things we should be teaching the next generation, and be learning ourselves, rarely are. In my view as a school district curriculum leader, the basic skills are not complete unless we include mindfulness among those skills. In that effort, Dr. Saz shows us the way."

—**Dave Del Gardo**, retired teacher, Cloverdale, CA; former superintendent of curriculum instruction, Eureka Union School District, Granite Bay, CA

"*Practical Mindfulness* is the perfect name for Dr. Sazima's easy-to-follow guide for mindful practice. Educators will be able to share and enjoy the mindful methodology in this book with students of all ages. I have successfully used his methods with third and seventh graders to help my students feel more control of their responses and aware of their feelings. *Practical Mindfulness* is a great way to help students and teachers become calm, focused, and ready to work."

—**Jane Thompson Murnane**, retired teacher, Eureka Union School District, Granite Bay, CA

Practical
Mindfulness

Practical
Mindfulness

A Physician's
No-Nonsense Guide to
Meditation for Beginners

Greg Sazima, MD

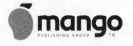

CORAL GABLES

Cover and Interior Layout Design: Jermaine Lau

Published by Mango Publishing, a division of Mango Media Inc.

For permission requests, please contact the publisher at:

Mango Publishing Group
2850 Douglas Road, 2nd Floor
Coral Gables, FL 33134 USA
info@mango.bz

For special orders, quantity sales, course adoptions and corporate sales, please email the publisher at sales@mango.bz. For trade and wholesale sales, please contact Ingram Publisher Services at customer. service@ingramcontent.com or +1.800.509.4887.

Practical Mindfulness: A Physician's No-Nonsense Guide to Meditation for Beginners

ISBN: (p) 978-1-64250-437-8 (e) 978-1-64250-438-5

BISAC: OCC010000, BODY, MIND & SPIRIT / Mindfulness & Meditation

LCCN: 2020949704

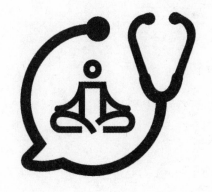

Table of Contents

Preface

This book is about making your life better. The solution is much closer to home than you might think.

In a broad sense, this book is about meditation, a practice that cultivates mindfulness: our innate, home-grown capacity for awareness. Improving our awareness makes life better all around, from handling the difficult stuff to embracing the wonderful stuff, and everything in between.

In a more specific sense, this book is about making meditation itself easier to start, stick with, and benefit from. Learning to practice meditation more effectively allows for it to become a truly valuable and regular "housekeeping" aspect of taking good care of ourselves and others, too.

There are a couple bits of irony in the title, *Practical Mindfulness.* While meditation can sometimes be portrayed in foreign or cryptic ways, our capacity for building mindful awareness through basic meditation is really not so far out of reach. It's more like discovering our eyeglasses balanced atop our foreheads while we've been rummaging for them in the kitchen junk drawer.

Similarly, the big "reveal" about the benefits of mindfulness is not about any external acquisition of a favored, permanent state of bliss. The territory is not gained, but rather uncovered: mindfulness illuminates and examines a true interior "home" of mind.

I can claim a deep understanding of medical and behavioral science. But at my core, I identify not as a scientist, but as a teacher. My skill set tends toward clarifying and translating the complex. I have the good fortune of a career as a practicing psychiatrist (I'll get it right at some point, with all that practice) and an educator. Some folks—my patients—allow me to help them more fully understand their lives and relieve their suffering. Others—doctors in training—allow me to help them improve their approach to helping those who suffer.

My own personal story features an additional, unanticipated line item: cancer. For most of my life I've been living with chondrosarcoma, a cartilage malignancy classified in the (dysfunctional) family of bone malignancies. An annoying hunk of misbehaving tissue growing near my spinal cord was mostly vacuumed out from my neck in 1981, when I was nineteen. The bratty rump of remaining tumor left behind, deemed too surgically risky to excise fully, sat quietly sulking for almost thirty years, then woke up tantruming as a more aggressive thing in 2010. It's required multiple surgeries and radiation treatments since.

I've subsequently had a crash course in applying my meditation skills to manage pain and uncertainty in the midst of a full plate of mid-life roles—as a (slightly glowing) patient, spouse, parent, doctor, and teacher. Meditation has been indispensable as a coping strategy and a rescue tactic for handling some overwhelming moments in that challenge. With my malignancy now in sustained (fingers crossed!) "neutral," my own practice has shifted—from managing acute suffering and the prospect of death, to opening with gratitude to a fresh lease on life. My path feels a bit like a second doctorate I've been completing, with a meditation cushion replacing the white coat, or couch.

This particular life course can cultivate in a shrink, or at least this one, a passion to examine the experience and share what I've learned. It feels like a kind of empathic duty, a compassionate act. Borne from those intentions, I've pulled together leading-edge ideas in several areas of inquiry—psychology, evolutionary biology, and, surprise, a bit of quantum physics—and my own expertise as doctor, teacher, and sufferer, to illustrate a better way of approaching this precious but unpredictable human experience of life.

Me and My Cushion: A Brief History

My first taste of meditation came a little later than one might expect.

Like most psychiatric trainees in the late 1980s, I was immersed in a profession in the midst of an identity crisis: psychotherapy and medication treatments battling for primacy. Neurobiologists and drug companies moved in with the heavy artillery—molecules, money, and marketing—aiming to transform the treatment of psychological suffering. Psychoanalysts, with their favored exploration of the subjective mind—of unconscious conflict, of oedipal complexes and funny, asymmetrical couches—were being unceremoniously nudged offstage, urged to retire to history's dustbin alongside the Betamax and the cotton gin.

Psychiatric training programs and their trainees like me were stuck in the middle. My own training program at the University of Connecticut, proudly rooted in psychodynamics, handled the dizzying shift decently well for us newbie shrinks. It grounded us in the potent value of talk therapy while making room for solid training in the burgeoning "armamentarium" of medication treatments for depression, anxiety, psychosis, and other maladies of the mind.

That rococo[1] term "armamentarium" is not my (only) lame attempt to wow you with my thesaurus dexterity. It was and still is routinely used at psychiatric conferences to refer to the varieties of neurochemical additives at our clinical disposal. It has always struck me as oddly militaristic, as if psychiatrists are going to war with malevolent neurons. Yet the alternative, psychoanalytic model has had its own war-games attitude and lingo, often viewing the mind as a battlefield

---

1   I just baroque the thesaurus with that term. Sacré bleu!

of secret "defenses" to overcome and "resistances" to confront. While the two sides wrestled over the contents of skulls—molecules and receptors versus mother-blaming and penis-envying—I'd always had a sense that the sufferer's own role in the process seemed to be left on the sidelines by both armies.

Education about stress management techniques and tools was mostly absent in traditional psychiatric training in the '80s. As I subsequently launched a private psychiatric practice, I routinely encountered individuals hungry to be collaborators in their treatment. I wondered: how might the individual be armed—um, outfitted—with some tools to participate in the process of reducing their own suffering? It made sense to me that cultivating a mind that adapts and works toward health and fulfillment might be more complete, more holistic than the reactive, pathology-based model of medical "combat." The ethic of the primary care training program I was a faculty member of, and the inevitable influence of my lovely bride, an excellent family doc herself, have also shaped my outlook: building a cooperative relationship with patients in not only treating suffering but in promoting health. It's about open minds, hearts, and communication, and not so much about flak jackets and "ammo."

In working to build on but also transcend the "battlefield" aspects of psychiatry, I dove into incorporating basic self-help techniques such as relaxation breathing and progressive muscle relaxation. That led me to a broader study of meditation and other mindfulness practices. Mindfulness has its roots in Eastern wisdom traditions developed three millennia ago; Western cultivation of those roots in contemporary healthcare has advanced more recently by the good work of Herbert Benson, Jon Kabat-Zinn, and many others in the last thirty-plus years. I was excited to apply what I was learning in my clinical and teaching jobs.

In our Family Medicine Residency outpatient clinic in San Jose, my colleagues and I noticed that a subset of patients with chronic illnesses seemed more routinely stuck in poor health, requiring more frequent clinic visits and after-hours emergency care, and yet seeming no more healthy for all that effort.

In 1998, we constructed a project that invited select patients into an eight-week class that taught basic breath meditation along with other self-help tactics. The participants quickly and clearly benefitted; within a few months most became more self-directed and adaptive, needed fewer clinic visits and after-hours services, and reported feeling better physically—as well as better about themselves—despite their medical burdens.

I was truly encouraged by the success of these patients as they used some basic interior skills to attend to, monitor, and often reduce their inner discomfort, even as I still harbored some science-bred skepticism. But these mindfulness-based practices were low-cost, had few side effects, and were effective against the sense of helplessness that often rides along with chronic states of suffering. The initial project became a model for weaving these powerful tools into programming for other specific groups: patients with hypertension, diabetes, and chronic pain.

This work also generated a personal passion to cultivate my own meditative practice. I found a teacher, a neurofeedback clinician and therapist himself, who also happened to have deep knowledge of meditative practices from his own Buddhist study of over forty years. He "got" me and my medical mindset.

My interest in incorporating other modes of understanding consciousness pushed me into inhaling the works of a variety of thinkers on the topic, from East and West: Ken Wilber, Steven Batchelor, Ken McLeod, Joseph Chilton Pearce, Jon Kabat-Zinn, Mark Epstein, Thích Nhất Hạnh, Pema Chodron, Dan Siegel, B.

Alan Wallace, and Daniel Dennett, among many. Bits and pieces of their thinking informed my own view and have influenced my own clinical and volunteer work through the 2000s. This work included training my patients in meditation as a "booster" to medications and/or talk therapy, leading group seminars on basic meditation, and a developing a curriculum for local elementary school children called *123 Focus* that has fostered meditation training alongside their phonics and juice boxes. Talk about baby steps!

For the last decade, my medical crisis put my meditation practice to a stark, personal test. I'm now managing both the blessing of a sustained remission of the cancer (hurray, radiation!) and a somewhat disabling syndrome, dysautonomia, caused by that treatment sautéing my spinal cord a bit (boo, radiation!...but, hurray, radiation!)

I've leaned on many of the tactics found in this book to make it through my own intense moments of suffering, not to mention the overhanging dread of recurrence, loss, and the impact of the whole #$%&*$^% drama on my loved ones and patients. Life has become a master class in walking the talk. It's also spurred me to consolidate what I've learned into the book you're reading.

You can use what I've learned to transform your own life by attending more closely to your interior experiences. You can transform. I have, a little (there's some narcissism for you...covered just ahead!), and have helped others in my work over the years. I've laid out the practices as practically as I can, using secular metaphors to reduce obstacles in building this interior skill set of mindfulness. If you've been curious about mindfulness and are looking for that kind of informal, accessible way into the practice, this is your book.

Mindfulness has a special benefit for those wrestling with medical illness, emotional suffering, and the stresses of learning. If a health professional, a teacher, or a caretaker has recommended this book to you, please thank them—this is your book too.

If you are one of those health professionals, teachers, or caretakers, thanks! And this is your book, too. Please take a peek at the Appendix that concludes the book, which provides an approach to teaching your patients and students basic breath meditation. I include this "spread the word" additional material not only to ultimately put myself (gratefully) out of a job, but to show my surgical colleagues that not all appendices require removal.

The result I intend for any and all readers is a wise, more self-aware, and compassionate way of living. In my view, that's the best way we can use this birthright, this precious human privilege of mindfulness.

What Kind of Book, Now?

Mindfulness, you say? Is this a way of slipping you, gentle reader, some cosmic spinach wrapped in a candy-coated shell? Lots of self-help resources are out there on the topic from bright and well-meaning experts. Many of them are, unfortunately, also laced with a confounding lexicon of psychobabble, New Age buzzwords, and other elaborations. My late father-in-law, a lovely and pretty self-aware guy by the way, would kindly refer to this tendency by the term, "frou-frou." Wikipedia tells me that's a French-derived expression for upholstered fabric elaborations on apparel and draperies. Yup, that can kinda fit. It can reinforce a cliché of meditation as an esoteric and unapproachable activity—not a practical one.

I fret (that's frou-frou-stration, I think) when that gets in the way of the real power of a developing connection to a fuller awareness. But in working with the practices, I don't begrudge any use of a cultural "accoutrement," be it a rosary, a prayer bowl, or anything else that aids in the training of awareness. Frou-frou away, if that's your thing. Yes, this is your book, too.

Ever since Lucy the Australopithecus simmered with her grievance over chauvinism on the dusty savannah, and Piltdown Man[2] wrestled with his shame upon being called a fraud, self-help books have been a necessary, useful, but not always interesting resource. I hope to change that: a no-nonsense book on attention that, well, holds your attention.

We are practically home right now, already practically there. It's been there all the time, just waiting for us to turn on a light or two.

---

2   Famously fossilized hoax.

Just Take a Breath Already, Will Ya?

First, take a breath. A nice deep one. Try to stick your *belly out first with it, like you are filling up a water balloon at the park spigot on a summer's day.*

Quietly, now, so the pal you're about to give a surprise soaking to doesn't hear.

Fill your belly slowly, then up through your chest, expanding yourself, making yourself bigger with good, fresh air. You're an accordion in a goofy band, breathing in an old-timey, lovely chord. Maybe an A major seventh. Something pleasant and smooth that the regulars on the park benches could get up to sway to.

Feel yourself filling to the top—past your lungs, up your neck, inflating your eyeballs if that suits your imagination. Pause there a moment, feeling full of life, right now.

Take a sensory snapshot of that before you float away or consider making a balloon dachshund out of yourself.

Now, start to let it out. Slow as you can, like a little pinprick hole is the only exit route for the lively breath. Imagine it sissing out of your nostrils, out your belly button, out your backside if you want to add some raw comedy appeal to it.

Or be that accordion, breathing out a slow, resolving D major seven, a long low "ta-dah!" The grannies smile and feign an awkward arm sway from a long-ago ballet class. Thanks for the memories, they beam with their eyes, as you hold that note all the way through to a fully empty musicmaker.

Pause a moment at the bottom of that roundhouse breath. Now pull out to a snapshot of the entire you. Whole thing—toenails to scalp follicles. No deep critical analysis, just a quick image of the bag o' bones in between that last breath and the next one coming up.

There's always a next one, or you've got bigger issues than this book will sufficiently address.[3]

Now lather, rinse, and repeat a few times. Fill from the bottom; imagine that squerchy sound as the bottle gets filled up to tippy-top. Pause for a sec.

Then, slow as you can go squeezing it all out to empty. Then, another quick snapshot: anything different?

And...scene.

Still here in full, your very quarks nourished by a simple act of a breath, then another, then another. Boring, really. Yet, when broken down, certainly a passable little bit of cinema with its own plot, its own drama. There are all sorts of ways you can dress it up in imagination.

With the interior sensation of your squeezebox moving in and out, your awareness is also there, ever-present, shooting footage. You can telephoto in on the navel or the nostril; you can pull out to a panorama view of your whole landscape of experience—body, emotion, thoughts, even out past those items to the full setting you are embedded in: the immediate space around you, out to the city or area, even out to the whole cosmic enchilada.

This is, all of it, home.

---

3   Hint...call 911.

So, where's home?

We usually think of home as a place of safety and security from danger without. It's a refuge from the thrum of the daily activity and stresses that are an inevitable aspect of contemporary life. It's a spot to leave from and come back to: "home base" is what we called it in the summer evening games of kick-the-can we played long ago in my neighborhood cul-de-sac.

On an individual, felt-sense[4] level, what defines "home"? Commonly, it's the most precious thing we identify with: a body image, our occupation, a relationship, or a connection to our Spirit/God/Earth Mama of choice.

For many, the interior "home" is unfortunately centered on stuff outside of ourselves—*external constructs*, to throw some psychobabble[5] at you. For proof, we need only step outside to our backyards with barbecue stations that resemble election coverage news sets, kept pristine with nuclear-strength power washers to deal with the stray quark on the patio. Inside, behold our television screens the sizes of which would make a cartoon super-villain envious.

And if it's not acquired stuff we obsess about, it's our self-imposed dust storms of digital distractions: texters texting, Twitterers tweeting, Snapchatters snapping and/or chatting, or whatever. In goods and deeds, Americans especially seem to be desperately externalizing most everything to find a sense of "home" and stuff for it.

Home, Um, Deranged

I have (or do), therefore I am. While items and actions have their own innate value, it's amazing how many possessors of said items don't

---

4   As in, what your senses are yelling at you in this very moment.
5   Book club readers may wish to make a drinking game out of identifying psychobabble terms. Please appoint a designated driver.

really know why they shelled out the dough. I can't tell you how many times in the last two decades I've engaged in a (perhaps less snarky) variation of the following conversation:

> *Patient: So, I got this great new [fill in the blank...Land Rover/ jet ski/Gucci handbag/sub-zero fridge the size of Alaska/etc.] It's so great!*
>
> *Shrink: Sounds interesting. So, why'd you decide to get that? What does it do for you?*
>
> *Patient: (Shoots a brief glare of, "Are you f***ing crazy? It's got seven heated seat settings!") What do you mean?*
>
> *Shrink: I'm just wondering what the purchase means to you, why you got it now, your expectations for it in your life. That kinda thing.*
>
> *Patient: Well, uh, it's...[a great buy/what I always wanted.../the best on the market/my ass of a neighbor has one and I'm keeping up]. What's wrong with that?*
>
> *Shrink: No big deal, just wondering what it means in the context of why you're here in treatment. You know, what does it mean? Is it a need or a want, or what?*
>
> *(Note: I can be a real pain in the ass this way. Yet they keep show- ing up.)*
>
> *Patient: (After some hemming and hawing) I'm not really sure why I got this now—just seemed like I needed it. It felt good at the time, but I don't know now (and stifles, "And thanks a bunch, Dr. Buzz-kill!").*

I'm not generally out to shame anyone sporting a nice new purchase or appetite, lest I examine my own heart for envy at another's good fortune. Yet we often buy stuff impulsively, do stuff mindlessly, and feel stuff without much awareness or self-inquiry. We attempt to soothe a need or craving, not even sure what we're hungry for. This habit of spending our way to fulfillment (or distraction) has left many individuals deeply in debt.

Yet, still hungry. The unfortunate impact is that, despite all of this activity, contentment is elusive. Here in America, we sit at a mediocre nineteenth place in the 2019 Gallup Poll "State of World Happiness" rankings of contentment. Recent World Health Organization data ironically show that we do lead in another stat—that our rates of anxiety and mood disorders are among the highest on the planet.

Even with the mass of acquisitions and distractions we accumulate, most of us rarely ask of ourselves, "why this thing, and why now?" Does the possession serve a valid meaning? A clear path to contentment? Or might it only duct tape together a kind of superficially "fulfilled" home?

How come our home is never enough?

Let's revisit that different, more personal view of "home," the one I hinted at a few pages ago. This home that each of us resides in, twenty-four seven, is the place most of us locate between our ears: our own home of mind. It's always available for occupancy, always a place to return to and seek peace and comfort in. A comprehensive, deep familiarity with our inner "home"—with its sunny sitting spots, nooks and crannies, and boxes we think are full of old bills that may instead contain cherished snapshots—is a valuable thing.

Mindfulness involves attending to that home of our own minds, cultivating a clearer and more open sense of how and why we do the stuff we do. It's there, waiting to be nestled into. But for many, it's an uncharted place, a dull and dusty space that can't compete with the distracting dazzle of one's external appetites. Maybe it even seems haunted.

Discontent can have a variety of different causes, but here's a predominant one: in trying to soothe ourselves with "stuff," we ignore where we already are.

It's as if no one's home at all.

Lost in the Library

"No one home" can manifest in a range of ways. We may seek cover in our various types of thought—memory, speculation, analysis, even obsession. This realm of symbolic constructs[6] is a valid aspect of mind: it helps us prepare for the present and speculate about the future. But it can also be used as a hideout spot. To strain the metaphor, we may think of this aspect of home as the "library," and a common hidey hole for many of us, a place we escape to rather than living in real time and space.

Back in college at Johns Hopkins, they had a big, somewhat intimidating library fronting the campus, named for Milton Eisenhower. The "Milton Hilton," we nerds called it. This less famous, "other" Eisenhower, Ike's younger brother, was nevertheless a force to be reckoned with in his own right, as a college president. His namesake building is a remarkable thing; it's a huge structure, but with most of it underground—six floors of it buried in the Baltimore mud.

The world down below the lobby floor was an odd one. Sound was squelched by the building's entombment. The only sense of life came from the faint padding and murmuring of scholars and the greenish, evanescent flash and mechanical clanking of distant copiers. It was a kind of subterranean commune, with zealous nerds claiming obscure study carrels in the deepest levels of the catacombs. Some never left, I suppose, still subsisting to this day on vending machine crackers and copy toner. When (or if) these students emerged into day, blinking

---

6   Another "construct" ...bottoms up!

and discombobulated like newborns, they seemed unprepared to experience real life up on the surface.

We can echo this with our own interior home of mind. Fearful of what we might find with a broader view, we keep the lights dim, or even off. We may contract tightly around our thoughts as a defense against intense emotions like fear or anger. We can play "mindless," mostly tuned out to momentary experience, being vaguely present, but deadened to the world's full display, and obscuring our immersion in at the broader reality of life.

Or we can get so spun up into thought process—reminiscence, analysis, and speculation—that the experience of "now"—simply noticing gravity, the shoes on our feet, the wind on our faces— becomes the exception rather than the rule. These are just a few of the many defensive tactics we all employ, often reflexively. These maneuvers generate their own distortions and additional suffering.

My goal is for this book to introduce you, or perhaps reacquaint you, with your own inner, ultimately boundless "home." Mastering practical skills in staying more awake and aware, we can push back against forces of mindlessness that operate to keep us mesmerized and tuned out. Hopefully this makes a sufficient case for learning mindfulness for you, as it initially did for me: as a trainable capacity that yields benefits in managing stress and increasing clarity and wisdom in the day-to-day.

This nuts-and-bolts rationale may nevertheless seem a bit limited to some of us also drawn to meditation with broader aspirations, for deeper, more profound experiences of consciousness. Over the past four millennia, many individuals have experienced and reported spontaneous, "peak" moments of profound depth, unity, and belonging, and have strived to cultivate them. The road[7] to these "deeper dive" states has historically run through the world's

---

[7]   Often, a toll road.

various religious traditions, especially since the "peak" moment—and consciousness as a whole—has been poorly measurable and explainable in a secular, scientific model. Those limits often have driven aspirants, then and now, down the more spiritual/mystical/New Age "lane" in learning meditation. My own learning path has been a parallel one, gaining knowledge of the medical processes and benefits of meditation while abiding a deepening love and respect for the Buddhist approach through my vipassana training. There's benefit in both lanes; it's all good.

Nevertheless, there is an emerging case for explaining and accessing those deeper states outside of a mystical model. We can get there, too, practically. But we'll need to pull back our view just a bit farther and engage some slightly more complicated and surprising scientific stuff.

Quantum physics, actually!

A Quantum Curveball

Wait, come back!

No kidding. Quantum physics' framing of an energetic cosmic "field" mirrors a "field" of human consciousness as theorized in many spiritual traditions and, more recently, in consciousness studies. I'm by no means the first to point out these startling similarities among the quantum, psychological, and spiritual frameworks. Most of the legendary researchers in twentieth century physics, including the masterful Alfred Einstein, have puzzled over the possible areas of unity regarding quantum and consciousness. More recently, the philosopher and writer Ken Wilber built his entire career on a remarkable study of this mashup of science and spirit. Fritjof Capra's *The Tao of Physics* was another powerful effort to summarize and clarify the East/West resonance.

Wisdom traditions across the globe and human history have had awareness-building practices as integral to daily life, including Jewish Kabbalah, Islamic Sufism, Christian centering prayer, and others. Using functional imaging techniques such as PET scanning and fMRI, researchers are now able to witness the inner experience of consciousness, examining the effect of meditative paths and practices as they occur in the brain in real time.

Science and mindfulness can be seen not as at war, but rather as complementary. Both quantum and many contemplative approaches propose reality as a kind of endless cosmic stew of energy. Our individual experience of that "reality" occurs in the interactions of the ingredients in that stew—and our ability to pay attention to those interactions, to perceive and understand them.

That's mindfulness: a precious capacity worthy of being cultivated, and as valid a skill as walking and talking. And it's no longer a secret. Mindfulness practices have become a cornerstone of stress management in virtually every arena of modern life, expanding out of spiritual settings into workplaces, healthcare sites, schools, and even prisons.

Yet the idea of training this capacity can generate some skepticism from various quarters. Some religious ideologues generate needless, oppositional fearmongering, complaining that meditation practices risk a contamination to their value system. Well-meaning but similarly rigid New Age spiritualists can gum up this basic learning process with all sorts of rules and paraphernalia that serve as a litmus test for "legitimate" practice. And scientific reductionists may shoot it all down as poorly measurable, nonobjective, and thus invalid.

The great irony here is that those folks with rigid worldviews may well be the most likely to benefit from the practice of cultivating awareness, in order to temper their overreaction and to model some tolerance and acceptance.

The profoundly secular idea of getting better at harnessing one's awareness just makes sense, whether we use it as a way to manage our sadness after a breakup, to gain a better grade on an exam, or to reach out to a sense of the divine. We have the unique opportunity to take the best of both Western and Eastern approaches—both outer productivity and attainment, and inner contemplation and awareness—and develop our own healthy "toolbox" of skills for living fully in a busy, uncertain, and exciting world.

Time for a Field Trip!

While *Practical Mindfulness* functions as a kind of metaphorical "classroom" for learning about mindfulness, we needn't be glued to our desks for the whole lesson, hoping the teacher will get bored and show a video. We'll be taking a few field trips. You won't even need to tear your backpack apart to fish out that signed approval note from your parent.

Back in early 1970s, field trips in my hometown of Cleveland meant the Museum of Natural History, the Cleveland Orchestra, an occasional foray into the nearby "Emerald Necklace" of lovely, wooded parks, or a traumatic boat trip down the polluted, occasionally flammable Cuyahoga River. ("Water that burns" ...that was an interesting scientific phenomenon. They've cleaned it up pretty well since.) But for the purposes of this book, our "field" will be the inner landscape of the individual mind in the moment. There will be some classroom work for us, prior to scrambling for a seat next to the cool kids on the school bus. But not too much, as I want to get you quickly practicing.

The structure of *Practical Mindfulness* unfolds in three parts. Like the breathing exercises to come (hey, foreshadowing!), the book takes three separate breaths, each one having us inhaling some knowledge, then exhaling with some guided meditation practices. Breathing in, we'll dive into some frameworks of the metaphoric "home" of our experience of mind, to give some useful context for the tactics and routines of meditation. Breathing out, we will pivot into specific meditation routines that build from most basic to more complex as we progress.

In Part I, we'll start with a wide-angle approach, explaining our places in the broadest, endless field of reality.[8] It's a perhaps surprising layout of the field of awareness for our observation, informed by both spirit and science—speculative but deeply interesting links between quantum physics and our field of consciousness. I'll briefly clarify the physics and trot out just enough history to give you hives, in order to help you see how these two approaches overlap. We could dive deeply into this in an academic way, but I intend to keep the plot more practical and conversational.

My intention is to get us thinking about our own individual experiences in a novel way—a fresh view that echoes the way meditation operates most effectively, without preconceptions. We hopefully won't get too lost in the tall grass, and we'll return to this quantum "big picture" in more detail later.

We'll then tighten the frame and cover the first of two basic maps of our individual "landscapes" of awareness. This one shows the varieties of stuff that populate the mind's territory, using some familiar categories—body, feelings, thoughts—and a less familiar one: awareness itself. We'll look at how some stuff grabs your attention more than other stuff, and what that bodes for our struggling-to-stay-as-awake-as-possible-to-the-moment-to-moment life.[9]

With one big-picture framework laid down—a map of your own perceived area, sitting in the endless neighborhood of reality, as it were—it's out to that field with basic meditation practices, the first

---

8   Whoa. Get ready.
9   Hyphens were on sale...

steps in meditating. I'll provide some preparatory tactical information around the mechanics of starting up practice: options on where and when to practice, routines to get going sustainably, and some common newbie pitfalls to look out for.

We'll start with the historically vetted, firstest and bestest object for our observation: our breathing. Breath meditation truly directs us to the very center of "home." It's predictably calming and easy to internalize as the default spot for observation. It's always there to return to, whether quickened by irritability at a long stoplight, frozen by performance anxiety in the middle of a business presentation, or forgotten in a distracting scatter of thoughts while on the meditation cushion.

Getting off to a good start is incredibly important, so we'll spend some extra time and care here. I'll provide practice scripts for this first exercise in training up attention to observe the breath, and to identify and manage the different stuff that inevitably pops up as distractions in the landscape of mind. It turns out there are lots of ways to attend to the simple action of breathing. Some variations on breath meditation that I'll provide will give you some choices to try out.

This first field trip also features...getting lost. And found again. For me, losing attention is in fact a feature of meditation, not a "bug," nor a failure. It's just part of the trip. What makes us get lost, and what helps us get back on track (hint...the teacher said to return to the bus!) can be a fruitful part of the whole venture. Right at the outset, we'll start focusing on the importance of this sometimes-devalued aspect of the practice.

After getting this basic sitting work started, it's back to school in Part II. We'll consider an alternative map, a variation based on how minds have developed over time and evolution. This functional, "operating system"(OS) map frames the field sequentially from survival mind, to interaction and relationship mind, to rational/thought/creative mind, and beyond that to deepest connections with the oceanic cosmos in which we all are dog-paddling, awake or not so much: we'll call it "Vibe."

With this second "OS" map in our repertoire, we'll head out on another field trip. These more complex meditative practices build on the basics from the first set that centered on the breath, which is but one physical aspect of the whole landscape. I'll provide scripts to work with in moving the practice out to aspects of the entire body, including working with senses and with states of physical pain. We'll move from that body-based practice to tackle feeling/emotional states. From there, we'll dig next into the tricky business of sitting with thoughts—especially in observing our thoughts without getting too caught up in more...thoughts. We'll focus on some special moments—like anger, craving, and readying to perform or set to work—that can benefit from some brief but effective meditative routines.

In Part III, we'll open out from the more individual-centered aspects of awareness training we've surveyed—our own breath, body sensations, feelings, and thoughts—to meditating on the whole field, out to the space around and outside of ourselves, observing all that ebbs and flows in the moment. We'll review some earlier content about that dual nature of our reality conundrum, how both quantum science and spiritual traditions nudge toward a shared conclusion that we are all deeply connected in and as a field of energy. That stance opens up a speculation—that we can attend as our usual, separate selves, but also may observe for signs and felt signals of that deeper connectedness. It's an admitted complex and controversial topic; my intent is to open it up in a secular, observational way: what might those signals "feel" like? There are some common themes that observers from all walks of life and periods in human history endorse, which I'll dive into.

Then, once more we exhale...into some final, admittedly more complex practices in dropping into those deeper states of awareness. This "observation of everything" also includes an emphasis that I believe is important but underappreciated: awareness of our observing capacity itself. Besides the field and its contents, we can and should tune into the quality of our own watching—a quality that changes, like everything else in the field. My nickname for this "watching of the watching" is *meta*. Get ready for a bit of meta throughout the book; it's important. I'll tie everything together at the end with a review, some ideas on developing and sustaining the practice, and an invitation to proceed further with meditation—into more subtle observation of our own personal patterns and reactions, and as a tool for deeper contemplation.

But wait...there's more.[10] *Practical Mindfulness*'s boffo Appendix provides some ways we can incorporate our developing mindful routines not just for ourselves but for willing, interested others. Yes, just like we teach our kid to ride a bike and even Todd in accounting to set up a spreadsheet, we can teach basic meditation to others. The Appendix is a shout-out to my colleagues in care—doctors, nurses, health educators, teachers, trainers, and parents—who can help their patients, clients, students, and kids learn the basics of meditation. Teachers across the globe are discovering how incorporating mindfulness into the process of learning lowers stress and increases success.

We can learn to observe everything in and out of our own "home" of awareness, without any other goal but seeing it better, more clearly, out to the farthest reaches, and deep down to the most subtle and tender places. Life is not always easy, is never fully predictable, and ultimately is about handling that uncertainty. But there are some pitfalls and patterns we absolutely can get more aware of and adapt

---

10   A ShamWow? I just knew mindfulness was helpful!

to via cultivating awareness. The felt experiences of living—lovely, neutral, painful, all of them—are best attended to in full awareness. Here's where we start, gain some mastery, and create a foundation for a life-improving routine.

Hopefully a value-add for this project in front of you is that I've personally field-tested the tactics thoroughly, having engaged the content and practices of mindfulness first as a teacher and psychiatrist, then of necessity put them into practice in a comprehensive way since, in my wrestling with cancer. It's not my style to create a memoir of me and my misbehaving protein, a "Wednesdays with Greggy." But where it can help illuminate and clarify an aspect of managing a mind in stress (and in relief and gratitude, too), my saga provides some material to share with you.

I'm hoping this will be a resource that will stick with you. I intend for the book to be entertaining as well as informative, not a substitute for Ambien. You'll be the judge: while a core attitude in awareness training is observation without judgment, it's certainly ok to judge here.

Uncertainty...of This, I'm Certain

A final word or two are in order around what to do with uncertainty. Meditation generates lots of it. So does life. Funny how that works.[11] Uncertainty in meditating reigns in small ways, like in wondering whether our attention will settle down on a particular sitting, or big ways, like in perceiving a vague, felt sense of connection and belonging beyond our own skins. Deeper speculations about reality, while rooted in ancient wisdom and bolstered by recent scientific exploration and theory, is nevertheless not absolutely clear or proven. No known yardstick or whiz-bang scanner yet exists to solidify

---

11   Not "ha ha," funny, but...yeah.

this stuff as a kind of "Truth" with a capital T. There remains some mystery about it all, and that's ok. It has to be, really.

But as you'll find out in a "street-level" way in practice: sitting with uncertainty requires humility. In the midst of a comfort in what we do think we know, it requires a concurrent, deep respect for the immensity of what we don't know. On the other hand, that's not meant to be a dodge, either. I wouldn't present this stuff to you if I didn't resonate with it and feel strongly that you can be helped by it.

I suggest an "in the middle" approach. You can preserve, but raise an eyebrow, about your current way of being and observing. You can also dive in and explore with curiosity a novel way of being in and observing your life.

Let's get started.

PART I

CHAPTER 1

We Can Always Change Our Minds

Let's go back to the park, to that first scene I described.
Whether it's a water balloon fight or a single breath, we commonly
observe any such moment by taking the stuff in the scene and holding
it as present, solid, and secure in mind. We sit in a chair now, and we
saw that same chair a minute ago. Ergo, it's a constant chair-ness...
past, present, and heading into the future. There's my car, just like the
last time I started it up; its car-ness was there before, is there now, and
will be there in the next instant. There's my nose, just like the last time
I scratched it, and my beloved, just like the last time we kissed. There's
my opinion on the economy, or jelly doughnuts, just like the last time
I thought about those things.[12]

Our sensations and observations lead us to an inevitable, "it's me,
experiencing this" conclusion. The stuff of mind—perceptions of
input, and feelings and thoughts about that input—appears to stay,
from scene to scene to scene. We sense, we feel, we think, and then
we park the results of those workings of mind in what looks like an
oversized piece of chewed bubble gum in the cranium, often with
little follow-up attention to their continuing validity.

Thus, it may be a difficult sales pitch to invite us to take a look at our
own active minds in a different light. Our usual way of experiencing
the world—individuals participating in events, occurring

---

12   Doughnuts should be currency, in my humble opinion.

independently in time—is actually just *a* way, but not *the only* way, of looking at the world and living in it.

Quantum science posits something very different about reality. We now know conclusively that the "stuff" of reality is *neither* flowing like waves, *nor* solid like a rock or a sand particle. It's actually *both*— quanta of energy in different flavors, endlessly morphing. That restlessness of form/not-form goes for everything, including you and me, and our minds, and our experiences. All is in a glorious flux.

We need some kind of name for this "stuff." I favor a nickname: "*wavicle*," as in kinda wave, kinda particle. This all-purpose moniker will appear regularly henceforth, to simplify labeling the stuff that comes and goes in experience, regardless of its form.

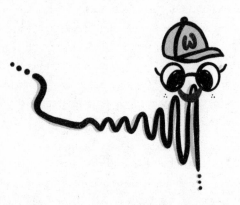

The Wavicle. It sounds like it comes in mango flavor.

So, try this: consider your mind instead as a cascade of experienced events, of frolicking wavicles in the landscape of reality. Observe that frolicking like one of those old-timey "flip books," where you flick through the pages quickly with your thumb; flip through fast enough, and the cartoon guy drawn on each page looks like he's moving, even falling right off the page.

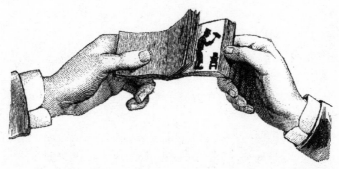

The proper name for this thing is the "kineograph."

We each attend to and observe what we can and own it as "mine." It's my moment, in my mind, in the midst of that broader landscape of happenings. Yet in each moment, so much more is happening than the one event or sequence we notice flipping by. Each series "captured" in our perception and then considered is actually sampled from a broader, shared field of energetic events. It's a cosmic wavicle park, with our water balloon-moistened pal, the cartoon guy, all past, present and future, all coexistent, all busy in the broader scene, all coming and going. In the park scene, some characters stick around photobombing every scene, while others are just making brief cameos.

In our everyday experience, each moment is like this: a "field" with happenings co-occurring, sometimes a lot of them, and other times not so much. It may be a direct conversation I have with a friend in a coffee shop abuzz with activity. Or it's a quiet moment at the kitchen table, sitting with my thoughts and memories of the day. Each of these moments, and all of the others in between, are "mine," but they are not only "mine." Each moment is also an interaction, a shared event occurring, embedded in and belonging to a broader field, an endless "ours."

In this endless, ever-changing field of energy, we ourselves are not only observers, but also participants. We're wavicles too, immersed in the field, our own energetic "selves" in wave and matter, altering and being altered from moment to moment.

That's the landscape that we are embedded in, and ultimately can tune into. It's admittedly a radical departure from the default way we generally perceive the day-to-day of life events, of an individual, separate-self outlook, versus how we operate in a broader reality.

If this sounds foreign, or even a little threatening, I sympathize. Most all of us live in a view of the day-to-day based in an individual "me," existing in time and space. We more or less have to. Imagine trying to explain any other outlook while in line at the supermarket.

Uncertainly, My Dear

Adding to our shared head-scratching about the wavicle nature of reality is the groundbreaking idea offered to us by the legendary physicist, one Herr Doctor Werner Heisenberg, discoverer of the "Heisenberg Uncertainty Principle." According to Heisenberg, nothing stays in place at all long enough to identify it and say it's "here," or "over there," at any particular moment. We can only posit a probability, but not any certainty, of something being located. So, ultimately, flowing and ever-changing is this soup of energy we all belong to.

We think it's "that thing," "there" and "then," but that's just the snapshot we each take in that moment. In the next nanosecond, that particular configuration of energy is off to the races in some new, wild way. Reality is a constantly shifting gaggle of wavicles, like butterflies already heading to the next moment as we arrive at the last one, swiping furiously with our nets and certain that we've finally captured it.

Complicating matters even further is one other deep development in our scientific understanding of reality. We assume we are objective observers of all that we apprehend, like flies on the wall, or like Marlin Perkins observing the wild wavicle from afar.[13]

Au contraire (there's some more frou-frou for you). According to quantum, the observer *always* impacts the field. In essence, no observation can be done that does not affect the setting that is being observed, at least a little. There is "no measurable reality *independent of the observer.*" If you sneak up on the wavicle, you inevitably crunch a branch under your foot and scare the damn thing away. Furthermore, this "never certain" thing around probability and observer impact is clearly a fundamental quality of all reality. A solution for this "uncertainty" is not to be found in more science; we won't somehow develop more effective wavicle nets to capture the elusive little buggers.

"I guess" is, ironically, the most certain statement we can make. Weird.

It would be challenging enough to pause here—at, "Ok, there's this reality of a field with actual stuff in it, but the stuff ultimately is changing enough that I can't take a completely accurate snapshot of it. And my photo-taking always makes some noise, which also messes up the shot, at least a little." Yet, this idea that the observer has an inevitable impact on the observed has an even deeper implication, one comically hinted at by a classic, if mildly vulgar, Zen trope:

"If a bear s***s in the woods and no one's around to smell it, does it still stink?"

If our observation of something in the field of reality inevitably and always impacts the field, it raises a radical dilemma: of whether there's an independent reality, or at least a reality based in matter, in "stuff,"

---

13   Mutual of Omaha's Wild Kingdom reference, circa 1967. As a side note, Marlin's sidekick Jim always had to actually wrestle with the damn wavicle.

outside that moment of observation—outside of that interaction of observer and wavicle observed.

Quantum infers that our experienced reality happens only as *a condition of our awareness*. An object in our awareness is not sitting around waiting for its close-up, like a languid model practicing a pout while we adjust the lighting. There's no model until we press the shutter button; and the model goes poof as the shutter closes.

Or, following on the bear analogy, if you're not there to smell the bear, there's no bear there. (So there.) If this is so, and over a century of scientific refinement of the quantum leap would suggest so, then the phrase, "we create our own reality," is not just suitable for dreamy philosophers and psychedelic research.

A Bumpy Reality

Let's linger for a moment on this idea, because it's big and a bit complex. We unusually understand daily experience as happening to a discrete "self" operating out of an individual "mind." We think of mind as a brain switched to "on," moving through time in a field of space, some stuff identified as me and/or mine, the rest not. We can call that relative mind, or *"mind,"* with a little "m."

Quantum, however, offers us a parallel, deeper reality of connectedness—an ultimate field or landscape of reality, with all aspects of reality capable of existing as wave *or* as matter—in shorthand, as those wavicles. That field never stays the same. It's unending, ever-changing. What could we call that? For shorthand purposes, let's call it big-M *"Mind."* The big M.

Quantum says that the stuff of reality is a soup that exists as wave and/or matter—wavicles making up an endless field of energy in constant flux. Observant wavicles such as us witness that field and the stuff in it. Our observed reality of that stuff *only emerges in the interaction itself*—wavicle bumping against wavicle, including the wavicles called you and me, dogpaddling in the sea of energy.

So, there are two flavors of reality we're concurrently entertaining. There is our separate-self, day-to-day, little-m "mind," built via wavicle bump after bump after interactive bump. There is also a parallel, big-M, endless/connected cosmic whole from which our bumps, and our separate-self reality, is created. In essence, little-m, separate-self reality is a moment-to-moment mosh pit in the big-M. No bump, no reality. Everything is deeply connected, yet our moments of perceived separateness are constructed with and by each interaction.

Lest you wish to draw straws or go to war over which is right or more real, let me suggest both are real! But they are co-occurring aspects of reality. Our day-to-day, standard, perceived world, defined by a sensed separation of self and other, is valid. Yet it represents a construction atop a deeper reality of connectedness: an unending, ever-changing field of energy...big-M Mind.

So, stop there for moment, and rest in that. Nothing stays the same. All stuff is in some flux, always. That's the basic nature of wavicles, of the ocean of energy morphing into matter for moments, then dissipating back into waveform. We can observe a hierarchy of complexity: interacting energy waves "crystalizing" into a range of forms from the simplest to the quite complex, then melting away sooner or later. It's a cosmic candy-making metaphor, if that suits your sweet tooth.

It's spooky in one way, but maybe something surprising and wonderful to embrace if we choose to adapt. The thorny conundrum to tackle, if we let this perspective have some play in our outlook about life, is, what do we do with it? How do we proceed with two tracks?

Kicking It, Quantum Style

So, dear reader, we move on to the central question: how do we hold, and live in, two views of our experience? How can we take into account the standard, separate-self, day-to-day of you and me in a "fixed" landscape, but also engage an awareness of the deeper reality of a fluid life of interaction?

What the hell would "living quantum" feel like?

The degree to which those interactions are perceived depends a lot on the complexity of the wavicles involved—especially the perceptive capabilities of any particular wavicle at the moment of bump. Referring back to the instance of our burly, lonely woodland friend, one does not smell the ursine caca without a nose, for instance.

I can alternatively imagine the vast majority of wavicles bouncing around like six-year-olds on the soccer field. They're a boiling hive of activity, reacting to each other in reflexive, but barely self-aware ways. Those wavicles that have some functional awareness to apprehend bumps, at a range of sensitivity from the merest electrochemical reaction of a paramecium's flagellum to the deepest, subtlest ascertainments of experience of a seasoned meditator, are truly privileged.

We humans have evolved the facility of not just a smeller and other sensory options, but also this wondrous attribute of awareness: an ability to be aware of ourselves and other wavicle critters in the field of Mind. We don't just bump up wavicle against wavicle. We can apprehend the bump and can reflect on the bump.

It would appear that very few inhabitants of the big-M emerge with this ability to reflect on oneself-in-the-soup, this exclusive, built-in luxury option to not only be in reality, and act in reality, but be self-aware of one's experience. But how do we really know? Humans could be in the preschool of cosmic consciousness, for all we know. Some higher mammals got it at a simple level; clearly my good old dog Gus seemed like he had it, sometimes.

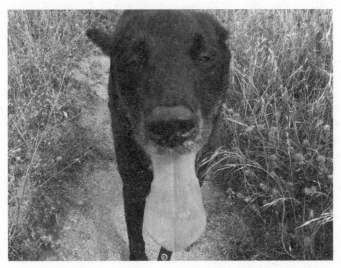

Gus the Wonder pooch, a sentient being.

Fewer still take this potential to heart and work to develop awareness as a trainable capability, as we would in hitting a backhand, playing a Mozart sonata, or running up a high score on a video game.

Take a Sip from the Firehose

Here's the good news: with meditation we can build a capacity of opening to the vast complexities of our minds. That's the prime focus of the introductory practices in *Practical Mindfulness*. The bonus value is that in training the ability to attend to that little-m field, we create the opportunity to open to a deeper connection. We'll cap off this book's practices with exercises that offer that opportunity.

Then, the bad news: the challenge of cultivating attention has gotten a lot harder lately. The sheer volume of wavicles in our landscapes has recently grown at a pace never before engaged in human history. For four million years or so, there was not much new and different in where we went, what we learned, or who we knew. Novel interactions with other wavicles were few and far between. Our DNA has been "shaped," more or less, very slowly over that long stretch of time.

For the last two hundred years or so, humankind has developed the ability to push the limits on our use of time and space. As a result of the technology of travel, many of us can meet people and interact in cultures that would have been out of our reach just two hundred years ago. With reliable lighting, the productive period of our day-to-day life is no longer limited to the time between sunrise and sunset. And in the past thirty or so years, the amount of sheer data that runs past us has accelerated in a staggering way—estimated at thirty times or more from the days of no cable and only three networks on TV. The myriad mass of wavicles competing for our attention will only grow more in number, kind, and intensity as we go along.

We certainly can choose to reduce exposure to the outside world and become more selective. We may shake our fists from the porch at the wavicles, telling them to get off the lawn and turn down their awful music. That is a valid, if only partial fix for "wavicle overload." But my particular intention here is less about how to limit what we're exposed to but what we do with that exposure.

If all experience is interaction, or bump, then understanding the bump is essential, and the cosmic market value of cultivating awareness goes through the roof. Awareness is the developmental tippy-top of reality as we know it so far. It is a capacity that can and should be nurtured and honed for maximum utility. The aimed-for result is a more supple, flexible mind's eye, one that not just watches the action of life but also watches the watcher, watches the watching. More aware of the interactive nature of experience, we stop white-knuckling the coming and going stuff of life as necessary for peace and comfort. Rather than holding so tightly to the stuff in our awareness for our security, we can work at resting in our capacity for awareness itself as our true home.

And, yes, we're practically home, right here. Mindfulness is a capacity that we all have. We uncover it, not acquire it. It's already there, waiting to be found, cultivated, refined.

Everybody Ready?

I've hit you with some admittedly dense stuff here, laying out a foundation for understanding our experience of mind immersed and interacting in a larger setting of energetic connection and belonging. Both ancient wisdom traditions and contemporary science offer a conceptual framework for this and a role for training up mindfulness.

From the spiritual, we are offered various ways of embracing a "higher power," divinity, and/or greater connection beyond and in relationship with the perceived self. Meditation originally grew out of this tradition as a way of accessing and deepening that relationship.

From the scientific, we have emergent proof of a basic energetic connectivity of everything and an unceasing flow of change of that energy, from wave to particle and back, in the ocean of existence. Our observation of experience generates out of an endless multitude of interactions; those "bumps" are registered and contribute to the construction of our perceived, individual selves. Meditation is a favored way to open in direct experience to both individual aspects of reality and deeper states of connection.

Whether one resonates with a spiritual perspective, a scientific one, both, or even neither, our prevalent perception of experience is mostly grounded in a separate, individual self. It's a self that suffers and it's a self that can gain some relief and adaptation via meditation.

So, that's the most familiar and sensible place to begin to train up this privileged capacity of mindfulness.

In this book, we'll start with a basic surveying of this landscape of mind and its occupants, for its own healthy benefit and to create the opportunity for that deeper dive. Running two tracks of reality may sound difficult, but with a plan and some guidance we'll learn to approach both. This practice—building basic, then more refined skills in awareness—offers immense benefit in both the day-to-day run of life as well as the deeper vibe.

Some maps of the territory will help. The next chapter will lay out the first of two we'll use. But before we dive into some conceptual material, it can help to get a brief initial taste of this mindfulness thing.

Already?

Sure, why not? There will be lots more detail on meditating to come. But just follow me here.

Take a moment, right now, where you are. If that's sitting, fine. If you are in motion, listening the audible version of the book, take a break and have a seat. Take a deep breath or two, then let your breath settle into its usual pattern without any extra effort or control.

Here are some instructions. Read each instruction fully through, then have at it. With each of them, make an effort, and realize that other stuff in mind usually, inevitably intrudes at some point.

> 💬 Close your eyes and direct your attention to that feeling of breathing. Don't force anything; just notice what breathing feels like—in, then out, again and again. Keep your attention on your breathing for five or ten breaths—up to you. When you either finish off

the number of breaths, or your attention wanders off to something else, you can open your eyes.

Simple, or maybe not. Maybe your attention stayed, or maybe it strayed. A couple of lessons can be found in this little exercise. There's a felt sense of our awareness as a capacity, as its own thing, aside from other aspects of our complex minds. There may be a recognition that other stuff easily competes for whatever is the current target of awareness—to highjack the mind into a thought, a memory, a sound, or some other wavicle of the moment. And there's a reaction that can come with the "pivot," when we become aware we've gotten lost from the intention of the moment. That's yet another intruder on the (not so) simple act of watching our breathing. Much more on that to come.

Here's another try with a little twist at the end. Read it through, then have a go.

🗩 Close your eyes, and again direct your attention to that target—the feeling of breathing. Just notice the in, then the out, and so on. After a couple of breaths, shift your attention to notice what in you is doing the observing. No real need to locate it or label it yet—just note that observing activity. If you get lost, you can return to some breath watching, then try to shift back to the source of the watching. Try for a minute or two, then open your eyes.

We're using the same familiar target, the feeling of breathing. The twist here is meant to show the target of awareness as being separate from what drives the act of awareness.

Ok. One more time, to reinforce the experience. Read through and then practice, please.

> 💬 Close your eyes, and once again direct your attention to the first target of awareness—breathing in and out. As before, take and attend to a couple of breaths. Then shift back to notice what in you is doing the observing. Rest your attention in that "observer" for a little bit. Then back to the breath as the target for attention for a few more breaths. Try that shifting, that back-and-forth between the target of observation—the felt sense of breathing—and the observer, for a minute or two more. If you get lost, just return to some breath—watching; that's fine. When you're ready, open your eyes.

The breathing and whatever that is in us that observes the breathing... they are different things, different felt experiences, aren't they? We'll work with lots of different targets for observation, inside and outside the body and mind. But here we are starting to gain a familiarity with that observing aspect of us. It is what we will uncover, return to, lose, and regain in the practice of meditation.

Ok. It's on to some mapmaking.

CHAPTER 2

First, We'll Need a Map

Make yourself comfortable...but not too comfortable; *the intention is training up attention, not taking a nap (though nothing's wrong with naps).*

Settle into a solid chair, every bit of you at rest rather than held in some tension or contortion. Stack your vertebrae like poker chips in a neat tower. A straight-backed chair works well; use a pillow if you need to bring your spine to a vertical position.

Feet flat on the ground—feel the soles of your feet pressing lightly against the floor.

Or, if you want to go old-school yogi[14] and use a cushion of some sort (jargon alert—it's called a "zafu..." it can sit on a "zabuton..." take me to your leader...), don't plop on top of it like frosting on a cupcake. Instead, try to sit more off the edge like a dandy's beret—tailbone up a little, pelvis pointed forward, weight more or less equally divvied out on a three-point foundation of your tailbone and the outside parts of each knee joint resting on the ground.

No need to make like a pretzel, unless you prefer that Gumby stuff— whatever feels comfortable and keeps you between the extremes of nodding off versus generating too much distracting physical discomfort.

---

14   Ol' Yogi U. Go Bears!

For now, better to keep your eyes at least little bit open, to stay awake and aware. But just pick a trivial spot a few feet away, whether on the carpet or low on a wall, and train your gaze lazily on it. You're not studying it for a test, but just parking your vision there in idle.

Now, consider a little starting routine I like to get the motor running. Take three successive belly breaths, focusing on making them slow and full. With each, a little interior comment to yourself:

BREATH one: "Here"—as in, settle yourself here into your landscape of mind. "Here" helps direct you from "over there," or somewhere else, like "I should be in the car now," or doing your bills, or whatever. Commit to this space, right here.

(Breath in, then out; note the feeling of the body at "breath all out.")

BREATH two: "We"—as in, "Am I the only poor, lonely schmuck trying to find some peace and clarity right now by sitting quietly? Of course not." "We" helps ward off isolation; someone somewhere on the big ball is working on this stuff, just like you, so smile. In a broader sense, "we" means "greetings, fellow self-aware wavicles! Let's practice!" That's kinda cool—reaching out into the shared soup by a single word.

(Another lovely wheeze, please. How do you feel?)

BREATH three: "Go"—as in, note your intention for the "sitting," just before you get to work. I know...is it really work? You'll see. Interior awareness building can be thrilling, or really boring, but mostly it's a patient, careful thing to do—and easy to get lost, even forget what you're there for. Setting the intention at the get-go may help you return home to it when you get lost in thought or feeling or sensation or all of the above. *And... Then settle into the breathing and its* *observation. Just let the breath be what it is, with no micromanagement. Settle back into watching what happens.*

My Very Own Snow Globe (It's a Blizzard in There)

First, here is a pithy summary of our thrilling exposition thus far. Reality is a big quantum soup of energy that coexists in wave and particle forms—those "wavicles." Our day-to-day, felt sense of going through life is actually a construction, embedded into and in relationship with that soup. As our experience of that day-to-day life emerges from our awareness of these interactions, awareness is a premium attribute to cultivate.

Let's look simply at "experience." What is it, really? Our friends Merriam and Webster[15] offer these definitions:

- Direct observation of or participation in events; having been affected by or gained knowledge through direct observation or participation

- Practical knowledge, skill, or practice derived from direct observation of or participation in events or in a particular activity

- The conscious events that make up an individual life

As these suggest, we can both participate in an event, a "bump," as well as observe it. Here's an example with some literal bumping involved. Greg's wavicle car loses its side view mirror, thanks to wavicle Greg being distracted by his air drum solo while pulling into the garage. Matter interacts with matter. A literal wavicle bump, right there.

---

15   That big, dusty book we used to look words up in. That thing you prop your laptop on.

Some wavicles observe the bump, if they have some degree of awareness to perform that feat. Greg hears the awful crunching sound and senses the odd shift in motion of the vehicle.[16]

The last point is the pithiest: these observed bumps can be reflected upon by a self-aware individual. Greg's dim-witted move, once observed, is then reflected upon—producing a series of secondary wavicles, including an increase in blood pressure, vocalized profanities, and quite likely a higher insurance premium in his future.

So, experience involves participation or immersion in an event—that's more or less inevitable, being in the soup of wavicles—and some degree of conscious observation of the event. Regardless of the observation aspect, just being there, immersed in the event, does result in some kind of effect. Even a stone, a wavicle bereft of any obvious faculty of awareness, does change as a result of a bump, say, of a rainstorm. The stone gets wet. A few billions of similar events later, a stone is now an eroded, weathered one, but no more self-aware for it. For those of us wavicles with more advanced awareness, we can attend, or play-act at being stony despite our more evolved machinery.

While simple enough on the surface—there's a moment, I'm immersed in it, and I notice it; there's another, I got that one—each momentary event, each generic unit of experience, really is a complexly constructed thing. We need to take apart that moment, that event, that bump. We'll start by conceiving a kind of map of the territory.

Let's start at the basics—what's the territory and its contents? For that we need some maps—in this case, sets of conceptual categories to guide us in our observation of experience. A common trope at this point in self-help books is to give a reader-friendly map of brain structures and functions. This is all well and good—the next

---

16   And yet finishes the faux cymbal crash with a flourish.

chapter will feature my own spin on that. But let's start elsewhere, by examining the landscape of our own subjective experience, with entities we can look for, recognize, and categorize.

We can picture awareness as a kind of field—observing oneself sitting there, taking it all in. We can notice all sort of things going on in that field, as we would on a nature walk: branches swaying on trees, the sound of birds and bees, the sensation of wind blowing in the hair, the smell of flowers, and so on. So it is with our own "personal" landscapes—there are experiences going on at multiple levels, whether we attend to them or not so much.

There are so many different ways to take a kind of basic inventory of the wavicles in the field—for instance, by size, color, by most intense to most subtle, etc. Here's one simple one: we can visualize five basic elements in that field of experience.

- There are phenomena of our **physical experience**, both inside our bodies and out
- There is also the experience of an **emotional "tone"** swirling around
- Also occurring, and usually garnering most of our attention, are **thoughts**
- While it can be subtle, one can become aware of the "**field**" in which all these phenomena are occurring—the "space" in the landscape
- Lastly, we can even be aware of our own *observing capacity*, witnessing this whole landscape of phenomena, ever-changing

We can think of the landscape of mind as a snow globe; the body, heart, and head are each prodigious snow-makers. Each of these types of phenomena (physical, emotional, thoughts) are generated like snow flurries, and the self is an observer of this ongoing, in-the-moment display. Sometimes things are calm, but the stress of daily life can figuratively shake the globe.

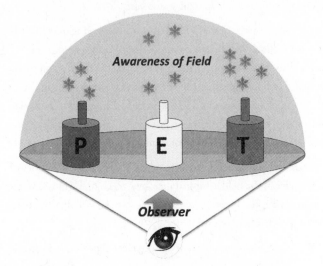

Your mind, rendered as a child's plaything for metaphoric purposes.

Hey, What's That Over There?

Let's break down each of these elements of the field a little more.

Physical sensation is a familiar category, with a range from the very subtle feeling of wind on the hairs of the arm to the gross, intense pain of a broken bone or burst appendix. For sheer nerdy purposes we can subdivide into "inside" and "outside," and the outside into the five senses. The interior phenomena include perhaps the most utilized one in awareness training: the breath, in and out, deep or shallow. The heartbeat is there, or if not, please stop reading and instead contact a physician or funeral home. We can notice muscle aches, the sensations of digestion, our sinuses clogging, a menstrual period about to start.

In quantum terms, looking at all experienced phenomena as signals of interaction/relationship/"bump," physical ones represent a particular kind of wavicle bump, often experienced as more or even the most intense evidence of interaction in the field—as opposed to more subtle apprehensions. Much of what we define as suffering is right here in this corner of the landscape, but so are the more pleasurable experiences, whether the taste of a fresh blueberry, the ecstatic sensation of an orgasm, or the satisfying deep exhale of a completed workout.

The intensity of the physical aspect of experience, in an evolutionary sense, is very likely protective for the gene pool. The pain generated by a leg wound is unpleasant, but those of our forebears who didn't have that signal to nudge some decent wound care were less likely to survive the thing and pass on their genes down the line. Yet that intensity can be misinterpreted. Like with a tantruming infant, a "noisier" signal isn't necessarily a clear communication about what's wrong.

The *emotional tone* in our landscape as we go about the moment after moment of daily life is another basic category we can build awareness about. Emotional states are actually mashups of physical and thought phenomena. For example, tight muscles, burning chest, and an explosion of "that's not fair"/ "I'm being messed with" thoughts in your head? Stamp that with the label "anger." The basic labels of those mashups—anxiety, sadness, joy, anger, etc.—are familiar and thus useful to identify and work with in awareness training.

In some parallel work I've done in teaching awareness practices to elementary school kids, I've twisted on the "landscape" metaphor to help the little rug rats understand—framing emotional tone as "weather." Nevertheless, it's probably not a surprise to note that there can be certain emotional states that even adults may have trouble identifying clearly or even at all in ourselves and in others.

For some, emotional weather is more or less an invisible wavicle critter on the range, even as others may scream, "Jeez, it's right there, right in front of you!" Academics label this problem "alexithymia"— an inability to identify and describe one's own emotional phenomena. It can stem from poor early learning in connecting inner experiences with their socially defined conceptual labels. There is a reason for that goofy poster in your second grader's classroom showing cartoon faces expressing different emotional states.

Positive emotions

ecstatic	blissful	confident	happy	curious
pleased	triumphant	attentive	self-collected	dreamy
peaceful	delighted	loving	sleepy	lovestruck
hopeful	sheepish	withdrawn	thoughtful	surprised
good	glad	proud	jolly	assured
bashful	idiotic	innocent	admiring	kind
adoring	calm	strong-willed	engaged	excited
interested	jubilant	inspired	grateful	tender
satisfied	phlegmatic	optimistic	meditative	sympathizing
relieved	determined	apologetic	indifferent	amazed

Negative emotions

demure	cautious	guilty	frightened	tired
envious	unsure	disappointed	hurt	bored
insulted	sneaky	discontented	ashamed	wistful
nervous	humiliated	weak	astonished	jealous
enraged	speechless	depressed	upset	lonely
arrogant	anxious	aggressive	eavesdropping	hopeless
gloomy	heart-broken	contemptuous	impatient	prudish
shy	repentant	grieving	resentful	mean
regretful	annoyed	suffering	obstinate	negative
cynical	suspicious	shocked	sad	unhappy

Find your face here!

Cogito, 'Ere Ya Go, or Something

The defining challenge of our physical experience may be managing and tolerating its intensity. The trickiness of our emotional realm is often in the difficulty in interpreting its signals. With the next broad category of experience, the phenomena of thought, our trouble is often around loving those thoughts a little too much.

Our thinking mind with the capability to generate memory (that is, thought phenomena "storage" of experienced events) and then reflect on and act on memory, may be something we take for granted as functioning humans, at least until we start to lose it. Yet it represents a truly huge leap in evolution. We can store events as memories and analyze them to speculate on future events. We can conjure new creative syntheses of those thoughts, generating more complex and powerful systems of interaction, production, art, literature, music, new beauty in the world and right at home.

It's not surprising, then, that thought, while one aspect of the field, gets most of the press, especially in Western Hemisphere history. René Descartes, the seventeenth century French philosopher and the poster child of rational mind over all, summed up things with the punch line from his famed *Principles of Philosophy*: "cogito ergo sum": "I think, therefore I am." He down-defined sensory and emotional experience outside of thought as physiological, even mechanical, but not an aspect of mind.

Western culture has mostly run with this approach, tending to overvalue that thought snow-maker in the snow globe of mind. "I think, therefore I am" is evidence of an identification with one's thoughts, rather than observing them as coming and going aspects of the landscape, like the weather. I've seen that wavicle in my field over and over; it must be my critter. It can be challenging for some to try redefining these thinky wavicle critters as events, as happenings rather than presences. But this maneuver can pay big dividends in stress relief, and we'll spend some time on it in our practice later. Let's not get too caught up in thoughts about thought; as they say in those TV infomercials: that's not all. The space in which all the phenomena of mind can be observed and contemplated is itself a part of experience and can be observed. In our camera metaphor, this is pulling from telephoto to as far back as possible, taking in the whole landscape display of experience—the details of individual sensations and thoughts but also the big picture, the space in which those wavicles are existing, acting, ever-changing. This felt sense of the whole field is for most a subtler experience—of fullness, of the harder edges softening around what feels like one's own body boundary, the sense of where "me" ends and what is "not me" begins. It's a lovely state to be able to open to, better yet to be able to return consistently to.

Also, there is yet one further, essential component of the field to locate in mind, or at least try to: what's doing the watching. "Field" and "watcher" are central to our ultimate goal of the experience of "vibe," and thus will get a fair amount of attention later. For now, I'll float the prospect that the two can be blurred into one—if not in rational, provable clarity, at least as a tactic in our landscape-based meditation practices.

That Was a Trip

This imaginative map of the territory of mind is one for the cushion, not the classroom. Here's a semi-helpful update of that last graphic, suggesting the pattern-set interplay of physical, emotional, and thought elements and the embedding of those features in a deeper field of energy:

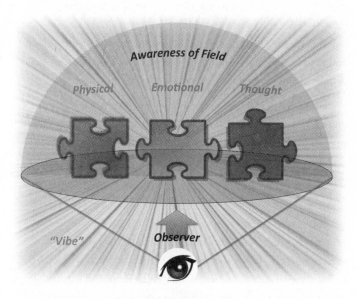

Your mind. Puzzling.

Granted, it's not a map of where the pre-frontal cortex or amygdala is, or how to locate a felt sense of one's left hippocampus[17] or any other funky brain part we can find in an anatomy book. While that information is helpful to researchers and curious thinkers, it's just not all that applicable or helpful in starting to grasp the complexity of our conscious awareness. It not really possible nor even necessary to note those brain structures as we sit in quiet contemplation.

Point, Please...

All of these phenomena in the landscape of mind are co-occurring, wild wavicles on the range. So, why pay attention to all of this

---

[17]   Sing with me! "Ohhhhhh, the amygdala bone is connected to the... reticularis pontis caudalis bone, the reticularis pontis caudalis bone is connected to the rostral ventral medulla bone, the..."

stuff? It's because we get in trouble when we operate on "auto-pilot"—tuned out to what troubles us (and why) in the case of painful experience, which often dooms us to repeating the troubles; and missing the good stuff that is going on all around while we're distracted and tuned out.

We may stay stuck in telephoto mode on one part of the landscape and tell ourselves a story about it, and, whether accurate or badly in need of rewrite, we likely repeat that story until the pages have yellowed and fallen out of the notebook.

Building attention is a little bit like standing in front of a wall of televisions at your local electronics store. All of these TVs are running—physical, emotional, and thought "stuff" in the field—providing information that would help us better navigate and even cherish our daily lives. But most of the time, we stay glued to one screen—usually the one with familiar loops and sequences of thought. There's absolutely nothing wrong with that aspect of mind, but it's best used as a one channel of our greater landscape of awareness—not like the ubiquitous *Law & Order* rerun, the only thing on.

While we can distinguish separate components of the full landscape, for the most part, the aspects of each element tend to occur as partners in pattern sets. For example, certain physical sensory inputs routinely generate an associated emotional tone and/or chatter of thought content. We commonly let these imprinted patterns run mindlessly and without inquiry as to their validity in the current moment. If left unobserved, these pattern sets can build up and run like viruses in the system—a root of much self-generated suffering. With awareness training, we can start to notice connections between the targets: for instance, a particular sense (seeing a flower or hearing an angry voice) can trigger quick connections to other targets (joy or fear, on the emotional level; memories of getting a bouquet from a loved one or of being yelled at as a child, on the thought level).

I'm reviewing and translating here, there's nothing new in this kind of "mapping" of experiences. Before the advent of MRI, PET, and other lovely engineering marvels that have allowed us to map structures of the brain (without the minor side effect of cracking open the skull and going ginsu knife on the contents), mapping based on observed phenomena of mind was all there was, dating back more than two thousand years. Check out the complicated and cryptic Buddhist prayer, the Heart Sutra, as an example. It lists phenomena of felt experience, including senses, thought, "eye elements," and "mind elements," directing the aspirant toward what not to hang on to too tightly in mind. The last five hundred years of Enlightenment-driven reason, however powerful, has not made obsolete this basic apprehension and comprehension of experience. The measurable and imageable glories of the current whiz-bang approach emphasizes the objective mode of investigation. Yet the interior/subjective mode—sharing and comparing common experiences of consciousness, however unreachable to date by a camera, laser, or radio-labeled molecule—still carries value.

Researchers in infant development recognize that we're actually born with a core potential for calm, open awareness. While this basic potential is built-in, because of conditions of modern humanity we start early in obscuring rather than cultivating this awareness. The firestorm (wavicle storm?) of new technology has only made the smokescreen denser, with TV, computers, and video games training children to accept distraction as "all that's on" and lose familiarity with the richness of the whole field. It makes sense to push back with practices that reinforce a fuller, more complete, moment-to-moment awareness. We'll sequentially "build out" from basic breath awareness practice to deliberately include the elements of that "snow globe"—

sensation, feeling, thoughts, and ultimately working on a "wide-angle" view of the landscape. Training in a more skilled apprehension of the field gives us a more accurate assessment of threats to the local self, should they need defending against. That training also gives more pinpoint clarity on what we can't change but instead need to metabolize, grieve, or adapt to.

CHAPTER 3

You'd Better Sit Down for This: A Few Preparatory Words on, uh, Sitting

Well, that was an admittedly elaborate setup. We covered enough quantum theory to give you post-traumatic hives from that college physics class. We postulated a parallel reality of something deeper operating underneath or alongside the day-to-day self. We've built an introductory, metaphoric map of mind to give it some context. Depending on your reaction, I offer either, "so sorry," or "you're welcome." But the success rate of just dropping onto a meditation cushion with some aspiration[18] but no real conceptual preparation[19] and hoping for the best is pretty low.

Let's reiterate the basic aim of this, or any self-help solution. Managing the experience of being human in this age, this dizzying moment in human history, is the essential task at hand. The sheer volume of various sources of information at our disposal resembles a roomful of carnival barkers, each clamoring for a fraction or more of our mindscapes. While for some, the speeding up of this conveyor

---

18 My spellcheck converted "aspiration" to "aspirin." A ghost in the machine?
19 Leading to a lot of perspiration. Or Preparation H.

belt of mind candy to be attended to plays to their strengths, for others, it represents a brave new world, and a stressful one.

And sheer content is not the only problem. In public media and culture, we witness the development and optimizing of ever more savvy and sophisticated systems of grabbing people's attention. Much of today's marketing to everyone, but especially to our youth, appeals not "upward" in human development but downward, to deeper, primal targets of the mind. At worst, the aim seems to be to exploit and destabilize the very human hungers and grievances in regard to politics, sexuality, appearance, and social acceptance that we are aiming to manage and model more effectively in our own lives.

The friction between the accelerating pace of input and the individual's ability to manage it—call that friction "stress"—has a profound impact on everyone young, old, and in-between. Rates of reported psychological suffering, particularly in first-world countries with the broadest access to technology, has increased over the last century, despite the self-help industry, Big Pharma, and first-name-only TV doctors. If unattended to, unmanaged stress can lead to a lifetime of increased suffering: physical and emotional problems, poor life choices in relationships and work, and unmet potential.

It's a battle out there, and the battle line is our attention. Attention is a tool, a set of skills to train. Using this training to manage an accelerating pace of life and its opportunities allows us to embrace change and its challenges. It provides some "Teflon" in the inevitable times of trouble in our lives and helps build healthy relationships with others. *Resilience* is an overused but useful term to describe this: the ability to navigate through stressful challenges and to grow from them.

So, What's Next?

Other than intentionally committing to meditation, there are few absolutes about starting a practice. The practice can be truly helpful even at its most basic—the simple, repeating practice of keeping attention on a wavicle of experience such as one's breath. That's where we start: this first of three sets of meditative training practices focuses on the basics of breath meditation.

The introductory aim is to create the conditions for a solid launch for this work to be successful and helpful. At best, it can become as routine as putting on underwear, brushing the choppers, or checking the email. Those of you who do not reliably wear underwear or brush your teeth may refer to Appendix XVII of this book for a list of haberdashers, dentists, and shaming moms in your area. There are some stage-setting ideas and attitudes to cultivate: an "A for effort" approach of both incremental benefit but also of inevitable imperfection, and "beginner's mind," an attitude of starting with a fresh set of eyes with every sitting, even when the current trend feels stuck in the mud. We'll cover tactical stuff about times, places, and spaces to optimize success and build a routine. As this whole practice can sometimes become complicated, we'll review the benefits of having an experienced teacher to help you along.

Then, to the cushion. Or the chair, or walking, or whatever, to the basics of awareness practice. No, it's not *the* "chair," though occasionally meditating may feel like it. As we'll get into, with any sitting, you work with what you get in that moment as an essential part of the practice.

We'll be careful and deliberate at the outset. We'll sketch out a basic sequence of beginning practices, starting with the basics of attending to the breath that many may already be familiar with, and working out from there via our basic map of body, emotions, thoughts, and field/watcher. I'll provide my own spin on them and how they work.

We'll deal early on with the central struggle of working with attention: the inevitable losses, surprises, coverups and where'd-that-come-from's that inevitably emerge from nowhere to hijack awareness. An intention and effort to watch one thing morphs suddenly into this whole other thing, hogging the remote. This is a facet of practice that is under-covered. Losses of attention are actually opportunities to learn, so we'll work on them, not to belabor or shame, but to use them productively. We'll emphasize an attitude of no-judgment readiness to pivot out of that lost state and step back a click to a broader, landscape viewpoint. My shorthand for this is *"meta,"* and it will become familiar with some explaining.

With some tools in "damage control," we'll proceed with some recipes for a couple of types of breath meditation. One can literally meditate on the heartbeat, the gut, the navel, or even the uvula.

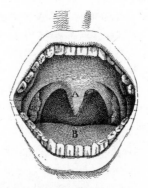

It's that weird thing dangling in the back of your throat.

Speaking of "body work," some specific exercises in using meditation as a tool in managing painful sensory experiences will be included in this section. We'll walk that out to full body awareness—for which attending to your lungs operating is a useful subset, if you think about it. We'll then march systematically through aspects of observing the other components of the "basic" map, including identifications of emotional "weather" states and aspects of thought phenomena that can flow in the field of mind. Holding that whole field in attention is where we ultimately will proceed to; Pokémon fans may rejoice as we not only working on identifying thoughts but also on pulling back to try to "catch 'em all" (as if we could!)

But let's not get ahead of ourselves. Anyone can plop down on a chair or a cushion, follow the briefest introductory recipe for meditation, and hope for the best.

(Spoiler alert: it's, "Step one: observe until you become distracted away from that task; step two: when you become aware of that, return to step one.") But that's, well, aspirational.[20]

The process can be a bit like dieting or exercising. There can be some difficulty and suffering in just getting going, and spells where there's too little linkage between effort and reward. For some, getting into a complicated physical position—lotus, half lotus, double secret two-thirds lotus, etc.—can lead to discomfort, frustration, and a quick exit from practice.

But the main obstacles to starting and keeping up a sustained practice are more attitudinal than physiological. So let's talk about issues of approach, attitude, and expectations, to hopefully pave the way for some patience with the process. Early on, it's about intention, freshness, and some humility—with an eye out for learning from the inevitable trial and error that occurs in trying to tame the wild mind.

Little Feat (or, Little Feet)

To the doing-doing-doing individual, sitting patiently in observation, especially of what can be some obscure subtleties of experience, may be a novel and uncertain pursuit. There are some comparable activities involving a bare opening to experience, such as a walk in

---

20   That's diplomatic-speak for, "good luck with that."

nature, examining a painting, or attending a cultural performance such as a concert or play, albeit usually with a set of expectations in mind besides, "what's this moment like?" As cliché as it sounds, especially as a cinematic, shrinky trope, it's "baby steps" at first that work the best.

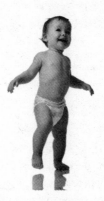

First you crawl, then...

However heartfelt the intention toward reduced stress, increased self-knowledge, and/or a deeper taste of undercurrent connection, a starting goal is, weirdly, best described as "no goal." A comic spin on this cryptic, "set a goal, but of no real goal" thing has been popularized by the meditation teacher and writer Sylvia Boorstein: "Don't just do something, sit there!"

That simple direction is more or less the totality of the practice in the Theravada school of Buddhism exemplified by the influential Vietnamese teacher Thích Nhất Hạnh. No complicated instructions from him: just sit, tune in, and see what emerges from moment to moment. There's a catchphrase for this direction, speaking to the (baby-) freshness of attitude: "beginner's mind." It's a reminder to approach each session of training, itself a novel wavicle bump to attend to, with a fresh set of eyes and unfettered expectations for what may emerge.

Child development specialists presume that an infant's awareness is open, uncluttered, wide-eyed, not yet running self-critical judgments of its state or situation. We can mirror this in our approach—like a mobile pivoting slowly above our wiggling, chubby little baby fingers. "Ooh, (maybe there will be) shiny keys!" I may be overstating it a little, but you get the picture.

From a quantum view, even the most expected outcome of any one moment, including one as structured as a meditation exercise, still represents a brand-new thing, worthy of an attentional approach that reflects it. "Beginner's mind" takes on even more importance in a long-term practice. It helps us work with the "seen it all before" feeling that can comes from familiarity, but can lead us to "play-act" at meditating, really being tuned out unless something new or surprising occurs.

The Other Met(t)a

"Metta" is a Pali (ancient Indian) term referring to loving-kindness, an "immeasurable," undercurrent, positive quality of mind—a good thing to meditate on, actually. But I'm referring to a different thing here.

"*Meta-,*" on the other hand, is a prefix indicating, "an abstraction from another concept." At least for our purposes, you may add the word "about" to a concept to get at the essence of it. "Meta-discussion" is a discussion about the discussion, an examination of the discussion. Ergo, meta-cognition is some thinking about the act of thinking.

And here's our specific target: meta-awareness, meaning one's awareness about and examination of being aware. In every moment, we are both immersed and observant. In the midst of sitting, we can become aware of the *quality of the experience of observing.*

Actually, "qualities" is more apt. One quality is one's overall *energy* of and for awareness. This sense of "juice" runs in any one moment from edgy and restless to slowed and sludgy.

Another involves the *clarity* or sharpness of the individual's focus in a particular moment. "Crystalline" as an ideal, but in reality, it's common to witness a spectrum from, on one end, a fidgety pivoting of the lens from wavicle to wavicle—the so-called "monkey mind" in Buddhist slang—to foggy or opaque on the other end.

It also includes the *stability* of awareness through any interval of time in sitting. This refers to the "stickiness" of attention—being able to remain on an object of choice without or despite the allure of other wavicles photobombing the scene, vying for the attentional camera.

Somehow paying some attention to the quality of one's momentary attention in the midst of trying to, well, pay attention, may sound like some personal screening of the film *Inception.* But it's valuable and nevertheless underemphasized in awareness training. Inevitable breaks in attention are better attended to, not as mistakes to clean up or bad marks on a cosmic scorecard, but as themselves useful evidence of where we are defended.

Early on, we need repetition to gain confidence in holding attention on anything. But as we go along, *breaks in attention are worth examining as evidence of defense*—distraction often being the shadow of something important, but perhaps difficult to look at. It may feel foolish or weird to "pivot into" the defense, to run toward the trouble, but that's often where the psychological action is. Some wavicles in mind are hard to hold in intensity; deeper levels of mind may step in to misdirect our attention so as not to feel discomfort.

Fearful mind can be like Wile E. Coyote,[21] dumping tacks on the road or placing arrow signs to nowhere or to a trap. These are moments, we'll learn, to return to an anchor or "home base," generally of the familiarity of the body and especially the breath. And then, "roll that tape again." Sometimes running it over and over may be useful, if it's not too painful to do, in carefully examining not just the objects in awareness, but how awareness operates, how it gets lost right at that very point—right before things go black, before attention goes south. Being aware of how awareness comes and especially how it goes— that's "meta."

Be It Ever So Humble...

You may have noticed my cryptic inclusion of the term "humility" earlier. Hopefully it starts to make sense now. We're always losing attention. But good news! We (almost) always get it back. It's impossible to be perfect at it, though one can find impressive poseurs at any meditation retreat claiming they approach that. Trudging over losses of attention can feel like reviewing a failed spelling test, over and over. "No judgment" as an intention is truly a necessity in doing this thing that results in so much apparent failure, especially in the beginning. Via a radical acceptance of "I guess that's just what's happening in my mind today," whether it's deep peace, a mind full of pea soup, or a hornet's nest of ruminative thoughts buzzing around, one learns the meta-lesson of watching our reaction to that ever-changing, mostly unpredictable show that we sit down to with each episode of practice.

That can sound demoralizing. Why bother with something that generates routine, inevitable failure? Here's the redeeming counter-lesson: even if the state of mind in clarity and/or stability may be a

---

21   21 It turns out "E" stands for Ethelbert. Really.

real crap shoot from day to day, the overall trajectory for just about everybody, if one sticks with it, is of overall improvement, on and off the cushion. Most folks witness a calming of the chimp-mind antics within a few weeks of patient meditation work. There are more and longer stretches of clearer attention in between the losses, and better ability to stay in clear observation of one wavicle in the field even as others may pull the camera off for a quick succession of shutter clicks.

There will always be days of complexity and difficulty, especially in times of stress. But the weather of the mind is always changing at its various levels, from somatic 1.0 restlessness, to 2.0 emotional roller-coastering, to conflicting or damning 3.0 narratives being blasted into the field, to the 4.0 camera getting foggy. Be a humble observer, whether it's clear skies or a storm front overhead. There's no real use in shaking our fists at the heavens for bringing bad weather, and it's a real distraction when we do.

You will absolutely need some commitment, effort, and intention to get this practice off the ground. Show up as an observer of the field of mind and see what happens. A steady, incremental building of practice works best. You could start with a commitment of, say, two minutes a day, growing eventually toward twenty by the end of a month.

Get a Move On

Some individuals by nature prefer motion to rest. For them, awareness training works better via physical activity. Truly, in theory, one can work to bring full attention not just in stillness, but to just about any activity, whether washing the dishes, sitting in conversation, or crafting an effective email to the grumpy boss. But I focus here on motion itself as the wavicle of choice in the field of momentary mind.

"Mindful movement" is a catch-all term that encompasses practices for which physicality is the wavicle object or "anchor" for the observer to attend to. Yoga in its many current flavors, Qi Gong, and Tai Chi are all examples of exercises in which attending to the sensation of motion and its effect on experience is the core purpose. Each has its own techniques, tactics, and history that I have no business attempting to teach you about. But there is absolutely a healthy benefit to physical movement of most all types. Our focus here is the particular use of movement itself as the meditative target for observation. The experience of motion is the wavicle for observation.

That can even be done with a simple, very slow walk with attention on the soles of your feet, or on the subtle feeling of energy in the limbs in motion. But it can look a little funny. A group of meditators on retreat engaging in what is generally dubbed "walking meditation," each engaged in a very slo-mo interaction with the earth, slightly resembles a scene from a zombie movie. But they're practicing attention and not too worried about the way it looks.

Bring an Apple for the Desk

Having a guide and support is always a benefit to learning meditation and sometimes is truly necessary. It's rare that the basic "model" of breath and body-focused awareness training can get a practitioner into trouble, with or without a teacher. There are even a number of smartphone-based meditation apps that run the gamut from very basic breath practice to a set of structured, sequential routines, and are a good way to get going for some. Trouble spots can sometimes arise in the deeper dive into reactive pattern sets of the mind, for which finding some live, human support and guidance can be very helpful.

The most basic kind of support can come from joining or starting a meditation group. Sitting with others in practice may sound daunting or goofy at first, but actually adds a sense of shared intention and energy that can't be duplicated in one's daily, solitary sitting. Time for comparing notes on experiences and obstacles is common in such groups, as is discussion of shared topics or books. Groups needn't be slanted in a particular spiritual direction. Many hospitals and medical centers offer training groups—some peer-led, others by experienced, professional teachers. Look around, taste-test a few, get comfortable.

More formal in the area of guidance is working specifically with a teacher. Finding one isn't too hard, at least in most metropolitan areas, but assessing the quality and ethics of the choices is not as easy. There are now lots of training programs popping up but no bona fide academic structure, as there is in, say, education or medicine.

Word of mouth from peers in a meditation group can be helpful. Understanding whether your own goals mesh with the teacher's is important; examples include more basic stress management versus deeper insight-oriented work, and a more secular approach versus one reflecting a specific spiritual tradition that you intend to pursue. Pick your approach and intensity and see if you can find a match.

There is also the important matter of sensing a good "fit" in working together, of personalities meshing. I'd offer a word of advice: humility. For teachers who trade on their experience to expect an "I'm the guru, you're the disciple" attitude, I'd run the other way, fast. Especially in engaging troubling patterns of one's own mind, vulnerability is inevitable, at times, and ripe for exploitation by teachers who may have tactical skill but their own under-examined ego issues. While sometimes the "tough love" of some constructive criticism or confrontation is necessary and beneficial, beware the teacher for which your repeated reaction is to come away feeling shamed or devalued. Little effective learning or progress can happen in that kind of setup.

Ready, Set, Sit

With some pointers in mind, we can move to the basics of the practice. But it is fruitful to keep these in mind and heart as we move ahead.

- *Ease yourself into the practice* with an emphasis on effort rather than some whiz-bang outcome as you start.

- Even if you've logged a thousand hours in watching the field of mind, groove in a reminder to engage each new session with *a fresh set of eyes.*

- Start early in entraining an awareness of your own mind's eye: *observing the quality of observation itself* (what I've termed *"meta"*). Be prepared for the inevitable shifts in that quality.

Go easy on yourself with whatever happens in any one session, or even a stretch of them. Be humble and careful with your *judgments* about working on this practice. It's a quick trip to self-criticism, to turn observation into a jury trial. Balancing that humility is some confidence, borne out from the individual reports of millions over three thousand years, that this thing helps.

Maybe sitting still isn't for you. No problem; try a *mindful movement* practice instead.

Like any skill, it can pay to get some help and support, especially as you advance. ***Consider a group or a teacher.***

And now, let us proceed to the hardware store. The nuts and bolts of basic meditation are next.

CHAPTER 4

Sitting: The Setup

Meditation's recent increasing popularity in our culture is a good thing. Maybe not so good is the caricature that has bloomed with it—the rigid, pretzel-like contortions, funny hand positions, and the rest. I think it leads to a distorted perception that some perfected posturing is the secret sauce for effective awareness training. Rigid recommendations even lead to just more contaminating judgment in mind: "Am I doing this right?"

There are no absolute "no-no's" in meditation except for lack of intention and effort. As it's about awareness rather than body form, meditation includes a vast array of methods and styles. However, there is a three-thousand-year history of meditation out of which has evolved preferential tips to optimize the experience. But if, say, a chair works for you rather than a cushion, great. If walking is better than sitting, go for it. Each variation can have some risks, as in lying down leading to the risk of somnolence. But if your back is a mess and you need to meditate lying down, that's your way.

It's the same with time. If what you've got is fifteen minutes in a quiet conference room at work at midday, use it. If it's two minutes at your desk before your classroom opens up, go for it. But developing a regular routine is the centerpiece for compliance. Find a pattern in time and space that works, then stick with it as best you can.

So, How Do You Start?
(And When? And Where? And...)

First, create a setting you can succeed in. Trying to learn to meditate in the family room with kids careening nerf balls off your head or blasting *Fortnite* from the big screen TV is not an optimal environment. On a trip to Kathmandu a few years ago, I saw a man meditating blissfully in the median of a chaotic thoroughfare, motorbikes and dusty '60s Datsuns buzzing by him and the stray, sacred bovine lumbering by, too. I don't know the Napali word for "chutzpah," but he had it.

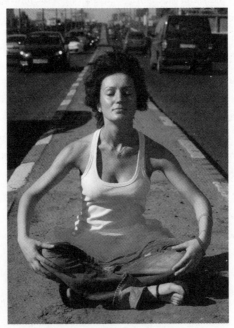

Don't try this.

For us mere mortals, it's best to set some conditions for success. Identify a regular, protected time in which you can be pretty sure you won't be interrupted. While there are no hard and fast rules about when to meditate, it's probably most common to sit in the morning. It helps cultivate that sense of "home" of mind as the rest of the day unfolds before you. It's not a bad idea to set an alarm reminder on your cellphone.

History is replete with reports of ascetic monks rising at god(s)-awful hours to get on the cushion. The Dalai Lama himself starts at three o'clock, the show-off. But there are potential pitfalls of choosing a morning routine. Some folks just aren't "morning people," whether due to their basic sleep cycle, constitution, or medical state. They feel less alert, prone to dullness or rusty joints. A little caffeine may help, but be careful about "overfueling" and causing distracting jitters and restlessness. If morning sitting just routinely trips up the attentional horse right out of the gate, try grooving in another time to practice.

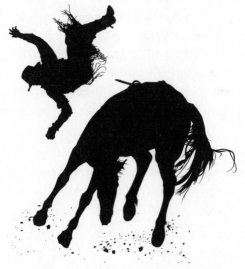

The mind has no force, of course, of course.

On the other end of the spectrum are individuals with minds naturally a-jitter with to-do's, uh-oh's, and what-if's flooding across the field of mind from the snap of wakefulness. They fail, it sucks, they quit; that's not a good outcome. So at least initially in starting a practice, if it works better to get a few things out of the "in-box," literally or in mind, before an AM sitting, try it, then pivot to practice. Otherwise, opt for a different, more fruitful time.

Others choose evening as an alternative or additional time to meditate, as it fits their schedule of available, uninterrupted free time. Basic sitting in the evening can help shake off the tension of a stressful day's experience. Evening meditating can also serve a good purpose in "metabolizing" one's experiences of the day: not analyzing them (that's helpful, but not really meditating), but sitting in the presence of those accumulated experiences—how'd they affect you? How do you witness yourself as a result? Are you different? What loops and habits did the day's itinerary get you hooked into?

The troubles with evening practice are probably obvious. It can devolve into nodding off. Meditation is an active practice of observation, even in the evening; fading to dullness and sleep is a different goal. On the other, simian side of the spectrum, an evening sit may not settle the mind full of chatter, but instead lead to more 3.0 itch-scratching analysis rather than the intended "bare" observation.

As with morning "monkey mind," this monkey should perhaps be attended to more deliberately at some point. But if evening practice just extends the day's tensions and makes settling down for sleep more of a problem, then find a more optimal time for your beginning routine.

My own practice has shifted with my needs. Early on, after fighting through the morning din of three boys clamoring for their turns in the shower and with the milk carton, I made the decision to commit to an earlier rising and meditating until the rest of the family arose. Age and medical issues have precluded the heroic/masochistic pre-dawn routine for a little extra shut-eye and a routine of an early-ish entry to my clinical office and practicing there. To be honest, I have a residual, "gotta clear my email box, voicemail, and faxes" itch that must be scratched upon arrival. A cellphone alarm prompts me to get my ass on the cushion for twenty to thirty minutes, depending on the day's crush of to-do's in running a solo psychiatric practice. I commonly add a briefer meditation—maybe ten minutes, sometimes a little longer—in the evening as a kind of "bookending" of my conscious day, as well as a physiologic exercise in attending to any physical burdens.

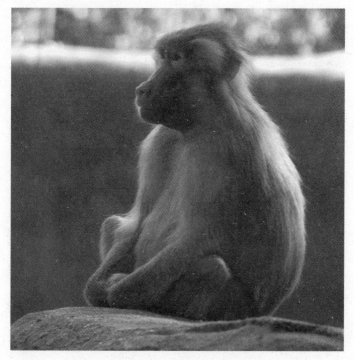

It can feel like going bananas.

As far as where to sit, that is also your call. I have friends in practice who plunk down wherever, and others who have custom-built meditating shacks ("zendos," in the Buddhist lingo), complete with sacred wall hangings and other aids to set an optimal setting for their own practices. It's your own preference, but there's no requirement to craft a temple for yourself unless that's your thing.

I'm personally not much for lots of trappings or decor. When I started out and plopped in the middle of my office floor, my monkey-minded state would swing around the room from branch to branch— to the desk I felt pulled to get to work at, to the door I could be walking through to get some java, to the clock on the table. It worked best for me to sit in front of a blank wall, lazily focusing my eyes on whatever funny-shaped, textured stucco spot I'd find a few feet in front of me. It admittedly looked like I'd put myself on "time out." Wherever you choose as the setting for practice, consider the impact of stimuli on your budding attention-in-training.

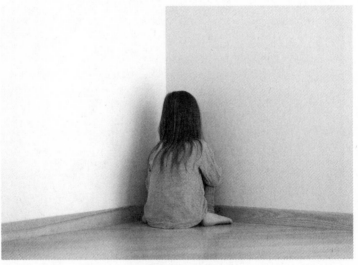

I guess I did.

Head, Shoulders, Knees, and Toes (...Knees and Toes)

Those with any experience in meditating in a group may be familiar with the variety of leg and arm positions that peers may exhibit. Full lotus, with both ankles crossed and resting up on the opposite leg, or perhaps touching the earlobes. Hands appearing to be making exotic shadow birds on the wall, or hovering in space above the lap, as if cradling a baby chick. Some others doing the palms up, "What, me worry?" position, perhaps channeling Alfred E. Neuman.

Ok, I kid. But these positions are culturally driven options. If you can truly execute the full pretzel, go for it; otherwise, the main aim is to create a seating position that is stable and upright spine-wise. From billions of aching backs in trial-and-error research over the millennia, the consensus is a stable three-point posture—the three points being the tailbone and the outsides of each knee. The tailbone is best elevated up a little, legs a tad downhill toward the floor in front of you, and spine, neck and head centered and straight up, to even the weight out and straighten the spine. My younger self with more flexible legs used to sit with a "half lotus," one ankle up and one on the floor. These days, well, nope. Back, neck, and hips should be aligned, shoulders relaxed.

There are different accoutrements to consider in finding an optimal physical position for practice. The culturally traditional, if somewhat cliché for some, sitting aid is a small, firm cushion, the aforementioned "zafu." There are pill-shaped ones, cylindrical-shaped ones, neat little jobs that looks like Pac-Man with a little notch cut out of it to tuck crossed legs into. Acquiring a dedicated meditation cushion isn't necessary, though. You can MacGyver it by using a couple of throw pillows, or doubling over a bed pillow, or whatever.

That little cushion lift helps set a sustainable, upright, dignified posture. Try sitting cross-legged without it; besides some fond memories of your kindergarten teacher reading *Where the Wild Things Are* to you, you'll probably need to curl your spine a bit for balance. The old saying goes, "sit like a mountain," not "sit like Charlie Brown's Christmas tree."

Early on, it's common to get some soreness of the pressure points on the outside of each knee, or cramping, or feet falling asleep. That really does improve over a couple of weeks of practice; the muscles and ligaments stretch out a little bit and the discomfort usually eases. One way to mitigate that pressure is to rest your cushion atop something else a little cushy. A small rug or blanket will do. The deluxe item is a larger, doggie-bed-looking thing to place your cushion atop, a "zabuton."

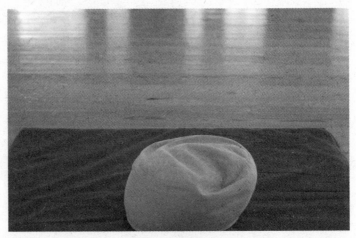

Zafu and Zabuton.

Still others with troubles in getting into a cross-legged position prefer to kneel; "seiza" is the Zen term for this position. This can be done simply by, well, kneeling. This semi-masochistic posture out of the Zen tradition, with feet inverted on the floor underneath the butt and the body weight resting above, can be tough on the knee joints and the heels that are taking the brunt of weight. Positioning a cushion vertically between the legs to take that pressure off the feet and lift the tailbone up can help this, as can a meditation bench—a forward-tilting horizontal bench about six inches off the ground, often with hinged legs.

If all the arcana about zafus, zabutons, seiza, and Pac-Man bores or distracts you, well, just sit in a chair, for cryin' out loud. You're working to find a reproducible, sustainable routine that allows you to be alert and not tend toward either snoozytown or an orthopedic consult. Pick a chair with a solid, flat-sitting base for the keister and a straight back; a pillow behind to lightly rest against is a reasonable idea. Both feet are best flat on the floor as the other two points of stability.

Hands? Try resting them gently on your thighs. Palms down, palms up, whatever feels right and nondistracting. The other common position is elbows bent, and hands resting one on the other in the lap. Sometimes I interlace my fingers, but for me, inevitably I start fiddling with my fingers, a little signal to me I'm restless or distracted.

We've covered toes up to shoulders; let's complete the picture. Eyes open or closed? My own conclusion is that it is preferable to start with eyes open. Resting the gaze gently on a spot on the wall or floor in front of you allows for all aspects of the field, including visual wavicles, to be part of the momentary scene of awareness. While eyes-closed can reduce sensory distraction, it can also tip the scales into feeling sleepy and less alert. While there are some practices that are usually taught to be done with closed eyes, and other with eyes open, again, try what feels right to you.

Breathing? By all means. Many inhale through the nose and exhale through the mouth, or all nasally, or whatever works if the sinuses are clogged. As we'll see, letting the breath fall to its natural, unforced pattern is a basic starter direction, after some introductory belly breaths to settle in.

Your mouth? The common instruction is a relaxed tongue, its tip resting just touching the upper palate. It's derived from yoga theory, the upper palate stimulating the sixth chakra, its meridian point, and/ or the pituitary gland. I personally find that direction a little picayune and poorly provable, but you have to put your tongue somewhere, preferably inside your mouth. Find what feels comfortable for you.

As I alluded to in the "meta" commentary, observing your own practice experience as you go and adjusting your spine position, state of eyelids, tongue placement, etc. via trial and error is itself an aspect of building awareness. Awareness of sweating these details a little too much (a kind of 3.0 conceptual distraction) is also part of practice.

So that's the setup. For you lovers of bullet points:

- *Routine and reproducibility* are key to make it become part of the fabric of your daily life.

- *Create a space* that allows for a minimum of distraction and that supports your intention.

- *Groove in a time or times for sitting that work best* for your energy and life responsibilities—but can allow for a reliable routine.

- There are a wide range of sitting styles, positions, and physical supports; aim for what work for you. *A stable three-point base*, an upright spine/neck/head, and a sense of sustainable comfort in the position are key.

I think that's the pith of the preparation. It's time to start.

CHAPTER 5

All Right, Let's Start Already

So you've diligently taken all of this preparatory advice to heart. You've got a quiet room with no expected interruptions. There's the zafu atop a nice rug to cushion the knees. Your cellphone timer is set to, say, three minutes. You settle on the cushion, wiggle yourself into a reasonably comfortable tripod, back straight, eyes half-lidded and trained on the carpet a couple of feet in front of you. You tap "start" on the timer. Now what?

It's simple:

- Step one: Observe some aspect of your current experience, whether a portion, or the whole of your experience, until you become distracted away from that task.

- Step two: When you become aware of loss of attention, without further elaboration or judgment, return to the task of observing that object, until you become distracted away again. And so on.

Thanks for reading, and good luck.

Nah. I'm back. Those directions sound simple but have some complex stuff embedded in them. What aspect of my field of mind should I pick? What's the difference between observation and thinking? How much distraction counts as distracted enough to stop and reset? How can I not be judgmental if I lose my way? Should I return to the same wavicle, or maybe pick a new one and see if that goes better?

These are common tussles in starting out; there are many more. Many newbies bail out because of early frustration. Some basic structure and direction to start is a good thing for the first timer and a veteran getting back to practice.

It makes sense to start with one familiar, reproducible aspect of human experience: breathing. It's one sliver of the physical category on our "fie" sharing airtime with the heartbeat, sensory pain, a gurgling stomach, or an itchy scalp. But it has great benefits as the tame horse to get on first before trying a bucking bronco. Attention to one's breath tends to induce a slowing and deepening, which naturally generates some calm. The improved oxygen transfer to your red blood cells that results makes your heart's sinoatrial (SA) node happy and slows the heart rate. That SA node, a complex hunk of neural tissue affixed to the heart, also sends back a message to the brain that peacetime is breaking out.

Besides that good physiologic stuff, the breath is a familiar spot to return to when you inevitably lose attention. It's often referred to as an "anchor"—the ship of mind can't drift too far away from that.

Learning to Breathe

Ultimately, we'll be meditating in "bare" observation mode, just letting the breath and everything else do what it's going to do and merely watching. But it's a good idea at this point to reinforce some full, deep relaxation breaths as a sort of "marker" of the home base to return to. It's like setting the anchor. Let's briefly review that breathing tactic.

Mindful breathing helps control vital, basic physical functions: respiration rate and heart rate. These functions tend to play off each other in feedback loops. The tendency of the anxious individual to breathe shallow, rapid breaths—"hyperventilating"—can reduce oxygen content in the bloodstream. The sinoatrial node we just mentioned runs the other direction in times of perceived threat. It will sense even subtle reductions in the oxygen content and send a message to the heart muscle to beat more rapidly and get what oxygen there is in the bloodstream to body tissues more effectively. That SA node also yells upstairs to signal alarm to the brain stem and its network. A vicious cycle of progressively rising anxiety can result.

We can reverse this cycle by voluntarily breathing slower, fuller, oxygen-rich breaths to full lung capacity. This simple but effective stress management tactic, the so-called "relaxation response," was made famous by a Harvard cardiologist, Dr. Herbert Benson, who first popularized it as an antidote to the fight/flight stress response.

For a moment, place your hands on your torso, one on your belly and the other on your sternum, and just notice your usual breathing pattern without trying to do anything fancy with your breathing. Unless you just saw a ghost or are standing in the middle of the interstate,[22] it's likely that your routine, resting breathing pattern is mostly shallow and experienced in the upper chest—mostly all we need while at rest.

Relaxation breathing, as was described in the vignette way back in Chapter 1, resembles filling a water balloon. It's how we breathed in our baby days, before adult cultural cues nudge us to hold our guts in. That's maturity for you.

---

22   Please put down the book and question your choice of travel.

Anyway, here's the recipe:

- Hand on abdomen, hand on chest (at least while getting the hang of it).

- Inhale slowly through your nose, filling your lungs on a slow count to two. Belly out first and then chest out to full.

- Hold the full breath for a count of two.

- Exhale slowly through your mouth on a count of four (in other words, twice as slowly as your inhalation).

- Rest briefly at the "bottom" of your breath. Visualize tension leaving your body as you exhale and gain control of your respiration.

- (Repeat the cycle four times, or more, if you feel like it; it feels good.)

This basic relaxation tactic has a simple benefit as a tool in calming, but also as a helpful part of an initial routine in starting any meditation period. You'll see in a moment.

HWG

We can meditate on any phenomenon of experience, or all of them. But three millennia worth of trials have pointed to the breath as an excellent "anchor" point to attend to and return to. The instructions are simple to convey, but often very difficult to perform at first. Starting meditators can be shocked at how much of a "blizzard" of discursive thoughts, shifting emotional states, and somatic signals immediately clutter the field of mind. One can plop down, turn on the timer, and promptly get lost like Yukon Cornelius until the mental blizzard ends with the bell, the meditator crestfallen in a sense of wasted effort, and nary a reindeer or "bumble" in sight.

While rigid rules can, at times, get in the way, there is benefit in having a routine in place. With apologies to a certain brewery's past marketing campaign, my own instructions involve three prompts just prior to starting off into wavicle-land to ward off the common complications of the practice: getting lost without our "maps," feeling lonely and disconnected in solitude, and working without some basic intention. Each of the prompts can be accompanied by an intentional, deliberate belly breath, creating some calm. The three prompts can be said out loud, thought about quietly, mimed like Marcel Marceau, expressed in semaphore, or whatever:

> **"HERE":** With the first breath, reconnect with one's mind as an open field with its components—physical, emotional, thoughts, the encompassing "space," and the observing self. "Here" roots yourself in the present place and moment. Some folks prefer "now" to "here," nodding to the momentary aspect of experience. Use what you like.
>
> **"WE":** With the second breath, note that one is not alone, with all of us in our own ways striving to reduce our suffering and find fulfillment. It's a good bet that somewhere on the big ball somebody is even practicing formally, just like you—a global network of wavicles in shared observation. Imagine that as you whisper or register "we." It can help along what can sometimes feel like a lonely task.
>
> **"GO":** With the third breath, set a specific intention and plan for the session. As our practices develop, this usually starts with a "warm-up" of watching the breath, then moves to observing other phenomena and patterns as we advance. But first, we'll start with watching the in and out of the breath.

My own sequence has changed over time, but always starts with HWG, then some basic breath meditation, pulling outward to body and then the whole field; then some variation based in what may be important to my practice at the time or in conjunction with my teacher; then a bookending of compassion practice (more on that later) and a capper of TWA (more on that, too, in short order).

Whether in basic observation of the breath, or something more complicated, remember that losing attention is inevitable. One can quickly shift from having attention wane to truly getting lost in the weeds—running a winding thought narrative or just zoning out into dullness. Setting a beginning routine, whether "HWG" or your own, helps with "returning home" and resettling yourself to start again.

Yer Basic Practice: Breath Observation

Settle into a comfortable position—cushion on the floor or sitting upright in a chair with a stable three-point base, upright and alert. Set an alarm (kitchen timer, phone app, etc.) for three minutes and start it.

> **HERE:** (big, slow belly breath, and...) Anchor yourself in place and time, and in the aspects of your field of your field of (separate self) mind.
>
> **WE:** (another big, slow belly breath, and...) Anchor out one step farther—you are embedded in a deeper, shared reality—not alone.
>
> **GO:** (one more big, slow belly breath, and...) Set a plan for the session. In this first practice, the focus is on the breath.

Annnddd...here we go. Breathing is an action that can be observed from its entry at the nostrils, at the back of your throat, farther down your windpipe, or down to inside your navel, as you witness your diaphragm moving, moving air in and out. Pick a spot along that route and rest your attention there. Try one spot out, maybe change it up next time. Observe it without judgment or analysis. Just be there and witness it.

If it helps you, split the observation into its component parts: the sweep in of inhalation; the fullness to the "top" of the breath; the sweep back down of slow release of air; the moment between emptying and the next inhalation. Or observe each full breath as a whole and count them: up to four, or ten, or your lucky number.

One other thing, right here: if you choose a lead-in with its three deliberately full breaths, that's great. But then, let control of the breath go, and let it settle to whatever rhythm occurs in the moment. If that's calm, so be it. If that's anxious and short, that's what you got. If it feels right to treat that tension with some deliberate breathing, that's a sensible act of self-care. But eventually move to letting it be, sitting as the observer, and minimizing your scripting, even of the breath.

Just a Moment (and Then, Another)

Jon Kabat-Zinn aptly defined mindfulness as "nonjudgmental, moment-to-moment attention." It's worth unpacking that phrase, leading with the moment itself as its own event, its own wavicle interaction. One thing that makes meditation training different than thinking is the "here and now" aspect of it, different from being enveloped in "there and then," symbolic thought. We're most aware of any moment when it is sensorially intense. That delicious arc just as the roller coaster goes from a pause at the top of the hill to plunging down the scree—that's a fully aware moment for most anybody who's gotten on the ride.

But moments keep coming—not just the high-def ones, but the simple, boring ones too, like a simple inhalation, then exhalation. This aspect of experience will become a felt, familiar, yet variable state as you move along in practicing it. How "right now, right here" am I?

Hey, This Is Easy...$^&^*(*)*!

Watch the breath cycle, in then out, right now.

Unless you are the reincarnated Buddha himself,[23] you will inevitably, at some point—a second later, a minute, or ten—lose attention. Something intrudes, distracts. A thought or a sensation or some other wavicle flutters by briefly or completely highjacks your lovely observation. It's "what's for breakfast?" or "ow, my knees," or, "boy, that author is long-winded," or something. Or it's a tune out into sleepy dullness.

What then?

Just as awareness inevitably slips away, there is also and eventually a lovely sweet spot, a pivot point, when the self-aware mind comes back online. We'll spend time later on this magic moment and some things to do with it. But for now, it's sufficient to be aware of distraction ended, attention regained.

Pretty much every teaching then provides the simple but power-packed direction.

"Without judgment, return your attention to the breath."

This is as opposed to,

"First convene an interior kangaroo court of your amygdalae, hippocampi and caudate nuclei, and proceed with a show trial for the crime of losing attention, you numbskull. Guilty!"

---

23   Wow, reading my book? Namaste!

There are two good reasons for this pithy instruction. One: such a convening introduces shame for losing attention, which is not helpful to the cause of continuing the practice and getting into a real groove. And two: that judgy narrative is just more thinking, an addition to the field. Critique isn't the day's plan, which is to observe the breath, not to work on a *Law & Order: Thought Crime Unit* screenplay.

In my curriculum for elementary school kids, I use the metaphor of attention being like a puppy who is trained to sit and stay. Patient repetition and kindness to the little pooch, most would agree, yields a better result than yelling or, good God, worse. If that helps, take a tip from the kids. Treat your attention in early training as little Rover. Be nice to Rover, and train that pooch kindly.

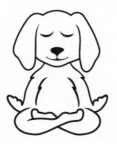

Works well for distemper.

So you try to sit in awareness, you do so until there's some wandering off to find a treat or to bark out the window,[24] then eventually a recognition of wandering and a gentle coaxing back into awareness while trying not to bitch (I know, too easy) at yourself for the wandering. Eventually, staying (present) gets easier. With that regaining of attention, there can be but a brief noting of the distraction—"that's a thought." Then let it go and reengage your intention.

---

24   Those of you contemplating peeing in the corner, find another metaphor.

But it's not a bad idea to briefly reiterate your "HWG" warm-up, especially if the distraction was dense. It can help to wiggle a little physically in position, reengaging the "here" of fuller body awareness. A quick "we" reminder soothes via the high likelihood that untold numbers of others are in their own ways also wrestling with their wild puppy minds.

Then "go," again—back to watching. Observe the inhale, note the top, watch the exhale, note the peace at the bottom. Proceed until another distraction occurs, and with it another opportunity to regain what was lost. Ultimately, you build confidence in a skill that improves with these simple moments of practice. Continue on until your timer alerts you.

TWA

Some folks pop right up off the chair or cushion as the session ends, like Fred Flintstone off the back of the Brontosaurus.[25] Instead, consider taking a moment at right there and then, and open your awareness out to everything. The lens has been on telephoto, clicking off shots of the breath when it wasn't occasionally shooting footage of distractions. Just for a couple of seconds, pull back to full landscape mode and observe your state. Check yourself out.

To make it a little more organized, consider a session-ending bookend: we can call it "TWA."[26] No need for belly breaths on this capper, but a nice way to finish.

> **THERE:** One brief re-check of your presence in body, heart, mind, and awareness, and acknowledgment of practice—there, as in "There, I did it."

---

25 This mindless movement practice well documented in the Yabadabadoo Sutra. Look it up.

26 Another copyright infringement risk...wait, that airline has been gone for years.

WE: A brief reminder of your contact, locally or remotely, to the self-aware gaggle of wavicles having joined you. Some gratitude may arise.

ARE: Open that lens all the way out—just let your mind be what it will be and observe how you feel. Come up for air, but with an observing eye as you prepare to head off to the next thing.

You may not need this actual structured prompt as you gain facility in meditation. As we get into more complicated routines in awareness, examining patterns, it can come in handy as a routinized ending, coming to the surface of your day-to-day mind.

Oh, I Gotta Remember That

This basic practice routine may lead some to see distractions as not just obstacles to become aware of, but as the enemy of a clear mind. But distractions inevitably pop up, whether attention is trained on a single breath or a broader view. That's mind (and big-M Mind) for you.

A common misunderstanding of beginners is that they're not supposed to have thoughts occur at all. In my classes, a few participants predictably return in the second week with a shameful distortion about perceived meditative failure: "I can't do it... I keep getting thoughts! I can't make my mind be empty!" This stems from a misguided idea that successful meditation means an emptying out of mind.

It doesn't help that Buddhism often uses the cryptic term "emptiness" to describe what I've rebranded as "Vibe"—a broader, open, felt sense of unity and belonging beyond the constructed self. That wisdom tradition uses the term "empty" to distinguish our separate-self construction—full of persistent, separate, "full" things—and the underlying, big-M reality of all things really just coming and going, not persisting and thus ultimately "empty" of any ongoing, inherent, matter-based "fullness" or "thereness." Yet the term "emptiness" can suggest that an ideal mind state is somehow vacant. Fear or utility over the impossibility of this supposed ideal can ensue. Where does the "me" go?

I'll tell you what I tell students: relax. Thoughts happen. We note thoughts and other distracting wavicles as they arise, and then "catch and release." Unfortunately, sometimes a thought can captivate and be the captor rather than the captive. We lose full attention for a while. Ultimately, we pivot back to the intended practice.

What distracts us is not necessarily "wrong" or "bad" by nature. In fact, it may well have meaning; a new understanding, or an old memory, or a wildly creative wavicle idea pops out. But what if the distraction feels important, memorable, not to be discarded? Orthodox practice recommendations generally insist on no stopping to take notes, as that's not meditating. Yet "gotta remember that" can lead to a secondary intention to memorize it while simultaneously trying to watch the breath. Good luck with that.

There are some options. One is to stick with the intention you set at the outset, and bank on the undercurrent, cosmic confidence that if it's important enough, the thought will arise again (and again and again). Another is a Post-it note and a pen nearby for a brief "note to self for later" can be helpful. But no novel writing, please—that's not meditation. The last suggestion is turning into the wind, so to speak. If an idea in mind keeps knocking on the door and interrupting, it may be worth it to switch targets and address the idea *as* the object of attention—to give it its due. This is not mean dwelling in narrative, but instead resting with attention on the idea and observing its effect on you—on body, heart, thought, awareness.

What's the Plan?

A regular beginning routine often involves starting with short (two to ten minutes) of sitting in the first couple of weeks, expanding the time out to twenty to thirty minutes or more as you get better at persistent and clear attention and become more flexible in pivoting back to the task after inevitable losses of attention.

With practice, you will become more adept at recognizing you've wandered off into thought and more able to stay in "bare attention" for longer periods of time. But this fluctuates with the ups and downs of daily life; even highly experienced meditators can have trouble with sustained focus in periods of higher stress, or any time. It's not a contest. The thing is to just go back to being in the moment. Period.

In this way, meditative awareness truly is a trainable skill, comparable to learning piano scales or hitting a tennis backhand. While any one session can be blissful or a struggle for both "rookies" and "vets," meditation does generally improve with practice.

Routine Building: Please Mind the Cough Guard

There are some basics that are central to cultivating a sustained practice, best organized in a reproducible sequence. Like one of those salad bars all the rage in the '90s,[27] most everybody lays down a bed of basic tactics. There's no slaw[28] against moving away from the structure when it suits you—it's your mind and practice, after all. But those chickpeas, canned beets, and whatever that vaguely bacony-looking, alien stuff[29] in the corner container is may not be for everyone's palate. I'll provide some variations on each layer of practice as we go

---

27   As it's been at least a few pages since a silly metaphor has been introduced, lettuce now proceed.

28   Oh, yeah.

29   Deep-fried wavicles = not delicious.

along to provide opportunities for dressing[30] up any practice. But a plan that is a little bit compulsive and routinized is more likely to be sustainable.

My optimal practice structure includes, at a minimum, these components, as you've likely already surmised from the past pages:

1. *Setup:* Settle in with a familiar setting, seating type, sitting position, timer, etc., some directed ritual that indicates to you a shift of mind from "not practicing" to "practicing." I'll reiterate that the aforementioned, three-wheeze "HWG" start-up, like the three sequential lights at a speedway track, is a valuable option, as its steps attend to three important elements of successful training But, of course, you could make your own. It can be a simple as "ass on cushion, now begin," or starting a timer, or a just a couple of belly breaths before settling into the session.

2. *Warm-up:* Even if you intend to proceed into any of the other sequences and options coming up, spending at least a few minutes on a basic "local" focus is helpful, even necessary. Starting off with the breath gives a diagnostic cue as to the initial clarity (sharpness) and stability (holding power between losses of attention) present. A frustrating blizzard of wavicles does necessarily doom you to quit. But a sense of the weather in the field may lead you to take extra time in basic practice before or instead of engaging further.
The warm-up can be breath-centered or extend to a brief, sequential body scan or set of check-ins with body, heart, thoughts, and field, "waking up" those areas of the field for attention. It's useful to then return to the breath and practice a little to shake the rust off around the familiar losing and regaining of attention. This can be timed (think five to ten

---

30   That one even I regret. Or vinaigrette.

minutes or so), or based on "feel," of being ready to move to the main intention for the sitting.

3. *Focus(es):* The main intention you set from the word "Go" comes here. That may be "stick with the breath," a sensible practice for newbies and veterans alike. Nevertheless, once a practice builds out to fifteen to thirty minutes, this can range from more granular work on the phenomena of sensation, emotion, or thought to broader patterning and/or other practices, all coming up.

   We'll focus first on practices that develop clarity about the nature of individual awareness. Part III's "Vibe" practices are qualitatively different. They can be the main event of focus. A variation on that is to spend some time on each in each sitting.

4. *Wrap-up:* This aspect sometimes does not get the, yes, attention it deserves. It is common in a formal meditation retreat for a practice period to start and end with a sonic signal, such as ringing of a bell or metal bowl. That can feel abrupt, like a nosedive onto the runway. In individual practice, you can land that plane a little more gradually. That can be a few entrained slow breaths, breathing out gratitude. For symmetry's sake, "HWG" can be bookended by a reiteration of the practice now done: "TWA."

Your skills at using time fruitfully will develop with experience. It includes judging the effect of periods of intense observation, gaining a feel for when to take a rest "back home" at the basic breath practice, and sensing when repeated and total losses of attention into chatter or tune out are evidence of a challenging "theme." Be curious and courageous when possible, but kind to yourself always.

Summing Up, What's Next

Let's close this how-to of starting meditation with some summary points to nail down these essential elements.

- Besides an optimal time and space for practice, get yourself into a *favorable physical position* for alert awareness. Use a timer to allow you to fully attend without clock watching.

- Consider *an introductory routine* that sets the field, connection, and intention, such as Here-We-Go ("HWG").

- Start with a simple but effective practice: observing the in and out of your own *breathing*. Pick a physical spot to count breaths, and/or watch each one as its own individual momentary event.

- Be aware of the *inevitability of observation being impacted on or even fully lost* as thoughts, sounds, or other intrusions occur. This is a natural aspect of mind; nothing to judge harshly.

- *"Pivot" back to initial intention* of watching your breath, moment after moment. If it helps, resettle the field with a brief reiteration of HWG.

- Be aware that the *distractions that generate losses of attention may themselves be of some import*. But the task at hand is not to "work on" them (yet); it's to stay disciplined on the intention of watching the breath.

- At the end, take a moment to pull back out to the field of your full mindscape. It may help to conclude with *an ending routine...* There-We-Are ("TWA").

- *Start at a pace that works* for you, a couple of minutes to start, or perhaps a series of brief, timed practices. *Gradually work on extending the time* as you gain facility in clarity and stability of your attention, as well as some tolerance of sitting still for longer periods of time.

● Develop through trial and error *a basic sequence that works for you*; this often involves a setup, a warm-up to engage sustained attention, a "main event" (or two) for focus, and a closing.

We're on our way. We'll get next into some variations on the breath practice, losing and gaining attention, and then the next steps in pulling the lens back.

CHAPTER 6

Lost and Found

Here—we—go: sitting here watching my breath...the *inhale, and pause, and exhale, and body sensation, and again. Rolling along for a few minutes, maybe I'm getting this thing down...*

Why didn't he call? He should have called! When he did that last week, his excuse afterward was pretty flimsy, so this just takes...stop. Aha...

Chewing on my date's behavior wasn't my intention this morning—I can attend to that later.

Reset: here—we—go...watch the breath. In, out, body, in...that asshole!

Alright, shake it off: in-breath, out-breath... Boy, my back hurts this morning... God, I feel anxious...what did I do? Was I too chatty during dessert? Maybe his cellphone died. I could drop by his work... Ow, my back!

Stop.

Mind is in the ditch again...this is hard!

Back at it: resettle in posture, here—we—go...

We've covered the basics of starting an awareness training practice using the breath as a first step. Hopefully the initial instructions have helped you to start up a regular routine. You've probably found some moments of success in stable, clear attention on your breath, and undoubtedly some other moments of mental blizzard, or tuning out, or some other struggle. That's all ok.

If you started with short periods, then built out toward ten to fifteen minutes or more, that's great. If you're taking shorter steps, that's fine too. Stick with it; pace yourself. It's better to slowly get the basic feel of "observe/lose it/regain it with care/back at it," than force yourself through some longer-timed period of being totally lost in thought or half-asleep, and ending up dazed and frustrated as the timer goes off.

Before moving to stretching out attention to a larger field, we'll nail down this single "object" practice via a couple of variations on breath observation as well as a different somatic target for attention. Then, we'll focus on the main challenge to master in the process—getting lost and found again.

The Basic Recipe

For completeness' sake, I'll lay out a thorough sample routine here—a familiar, reproducible sense of decent clarity and stability in attention. The subsequent variations in upcoming exercises will usually be embedded as the "observe" step, and sometimes some extra steps, in this basic recipe.

> 🗩 **Settle** into a comfortable position; set a timer if that's available.
>
> 🗩 As we discussed, consider this **prep, each with a breath:**
>
> **HERE:** (big, slow, belly breath, and...) **Anchor yourself** in place and time, and in the aspects of your field of mind.
>
> **WE:** (another big, slow, belly breath, and...) Anchor out one step farther—you are embedded in a deeper, shared reality—**not alone.**
>
> **GO:** (one more big, slow, belly breath, and...) **Set a plan** for the session. In this practice, the focus is on the breath.

- Begin by **letting the breath move to its natural state,** whatever that is and wherever you choose to observe it.

- **Observe**. Here's where your day's intention is put into action. It could be simply your breathing, or a more directed and complex target or tactic.

- Then, inevitably, you'll **lose track** of that observation. (It happens; that's mind.)

- Just as inevitably, you'll **find** yourself back in attention. When "aha, I've gotten distracted" pops back in, with a minimum of judgment...**return to the observation** of the breath (and then back out to whatever other wavicle(s) is/are the target for this particular sitting).

- If it helps, you may wish to **reset** with a move back to anchoring in the familiar "HWG" three-breath setup, then...

- **Back to the practice**, the next breath, the next losing, the next finding.

- With the timer signaling "time's up," consider the ending routine of **"TWA,"** also with three slow breaths:

THERE: One brief re-noting of the setting, and you in it.

WE: A reminder of your contact, locally or remotely, to others out there.

ARE: ...just letting your mind be, **resting back** in a more relaxed observation of the field. Check in with how you feel, briefly, then.

That's the basic structure—a warm-up in preparation for the session's activity; a patient, careful period of variable observation of the target; and a "bookend" reiteration of place, belonging, and this moment of directed observation, now completed.

Breath Practice: The Trey

The witnessing of breathing has been a central introductory aspect of any meditative training; in some traditions, it's the totality of the practice. I suppose that simply counting each breath as a "unit" could be called "one-pointed" practice, and divvying it into inhale, then exhale, the "two-pointed." Over millennia, many variations on this simple act have been advanced. In the Buddhist tradition, there is sometimes a fondness for a dizzy numbering of everything (eight-fold paths, four noble truths, etc.). From that comes a sensible, well-known twist on breath practice: three-pointed meditation. The three-pointer, or "trey," in basketball lingo. It is not terribly fancy, but a good lead-in to opening the aperture of attention out beyond the breath.

In essence, you may use the recipe above and plug into the "observe" step these three points of more detailed observation:

- **HWG**
- **OBSERVE** the experience of **INHALING**
- **OBSERVE** the experience of **EXHALING**
- In the **PAUSE** just before the next in-breath, open out observation to a *brief witness of the body as a whole*, beyond but including the breath (and repeat)
- **TWA**

And, of course, then you proceed to contract attention back to the next in-breath, then the out-breath, then another quick pullout to body, and so on. As with any meditative practice, expect some attention lost, then found again. No fretting at that drama; that's just wild mind doing what it does.

This only slightly more detailed sequence does a couple of good things. In adding "out to body" in each breath cycle, it begins some training in that "meta" observing and maneuvering of one's facility of awareness from telephoto out to more of a landscape view.

It also helps to anchor the practitioner in a recurring pivot to and check of bodily sensations. This shift to the body is almost always a good tactic when distractions come up, as those distractions often can pull attention "upstairs" into narrative thought loops and judgments. Having a regular practice in gaining familiarity with that body-sense will be important as we move into more complex practices.

Variation: The Two-Act Play (with Intermission and Applause)

For some speculative proof that OCD existed in third century BCE India, there is also a detailed sequence called "seven-pointed practice." Each segment of the breath path is subdivided into its beginning, middle, and end: three points up for the in-breath, then three more points down for the out-breath, then the body-sense check at the base as the seventh "point." What's "the middle of the in-breath"? As opposed to the, say, fifth point?

Frankly, I find this marginally helpful at best. I humbly offer, as an alternative, a slight variation that involves attending to each in-breath and out-breath as its own extended moment—again, to plug into that "observe" step in the recipe:

- Watch the whole arc of *inhaling up* to full-ish inhalation
- A brief *snapshot* of the lungs at some sense of *fullness*, and then...

> 💬 Watch closely the bellows **exhaling down** to empty;
> and...
>
> 💬 A **check** of the **body-sense** at the bottom. (And
> then repeat...)

Rather than "points," we're observing a process in motion to full, a pause to note, then a second process to empty, ending with another snapshot out to the fuller sense of physical self. I think it's easier to observe the whole flow of in, then out, than splitting it up.

We'll work going forward with pulling one's attention into the body—"filled with awareness" at the apex—and emptying that awareness out to the whole-body sense and beyond. Try it out like with the other variations, and see which practices help you fortify the clarity and stability of your awareness.

Like a Drum

While the breath is an obvious target in attention practice, it's not the only piece of somatic real estate that we can attend to. Anything inside or outside the body is fair game. We'll sit with emotional states, patterns of thought, and visual tableaus. One useful, basic target is thumping away in you as you read.

The heartbeat can be an effective anchor. The stilling of activity to allow witness of the heart beating can itself bring great calm, even literally allowing that beat to gently rock the body at rest. In an even more subtle way, we can imagine, if not observe, the subtle, doughnut-shaped electromagnetic field that the heart genuinely generates—while not as potent as a television's, or an MRI's, or even a laptop's, it's actually many times greater than that of the brain.

There's no trickiness to observing the heartbeat. While a doctor or nurse can hear a two-part "lub-dub," and maybe some other funny stuff[31] when using a standard stethoscope, the meditator generally feels a single beat. We can observe a change in the speed of the beat, and usually will notice some slowing as a general calming occurs with sitting.

The remainder of basic meditation rules apply: watch it until you get distracted. As with the breath, you make that pivot from "lost" back to "found," to awareness of that regaining. No time out in the corner is required, but just a noticing of getting lost, a nod to what pulled you away, and then back to the beat.

Stories from the Heart

Two of my own experiences of using the heartbeat as an anchor range from the mundane to the freaky. One may ask the question, "can I meditate with a chest cold and uncontrollable cough?" Well, yes, you can. But while it's perfectly reasonable to observe your own hacking up of a lung, that task can become frustrating and distracting. In those cases, I'll move the anchor to my heartbeat and observe its feeling in my chest.

We'll address using other sensory targets, like a candle flame or the smells in a forest walk, a little later.

The more riveting personal examples of heartbeat observation involve the necessities of a whiz-bang flavor of radiation therapy I underwent called "stereotactic radiosurgery." This technological marvel of a treatment directed specific and intense radiation at an exacting, three-dimensional volume of cancerous me. The number-crunching allowed for full-force photon radiation to target the center of that volume, yet drop off to near 20 percent a mere four millimeters or so away from outer edges of that defined shape to limit damaging the adjoining real estate of noncancerous me. It's like...no, it's, literally, a

---

31   Call your cardiologist.

3-D printing of tumor from not tumor, with a Chernobyl chaser. So it was theoretically a good fit for a small but aggressive goober in a tenuous spot, just like mine, approaching but not yet strangling my spinal cord.

The treatment prep first involved undergoing a mega-MRI of my neck with around ninety minutes in the tube to take one millimeter interval "slices." (The garden-variety diagnostic MRI takes one-centimeter image cuts.) Any extra bodily movement during that extended "playing dead" act could impact the accuracy of that resultant three-dimensional computer model, and thus could affect where Dr. Strangelove would later direct the death beam. So stillness was an ideal.

I started with some directed, controlled breathing to calm my base anxiety about the tight space, marathon length of imaging, and tension about my possible role in messing up the images. Yet focusing on my respiration—my rib case being the one part of me I had to move—was ironically raising my anxiety. My aspiration to control my inspiration and expiration was generating (wait for it...) desperation (and perspiration)—making me run narratives about the degree of 3-D error I might be causing with any excess movement. Of course, that only inspired me (hah!) to take deep breaths to calm down.

So, a different kind of inspiration was in order: I moved off watching the breath and moved to my heartbeat. This was made easier by the candy-colored earplugs provided to reduce the cacophony of nuclear-plant-evacuation-style buzzing and gnome-hammer-banging familiar to anyone who has undergone MRI imaging. The muffling from the earplugs tended to slightly amplify the cardiac drumming as it thrummed up into my head. I watched my heartbeat, with some checks out to body-sense (mostly, achy back on that rock-hard gurney). A weird place to practice; I don't really recommend it. But, yes, any moment can be a moment to engage in meditation.

The slightly freakier bookend to that "stay still for X-rays" tale came a few weeks later, when the actual treatments occurred—three forty-five-minute zap sessions over a week. It may be obvious that the necessity for targeting accuracy in generating the radiation "volume" would be wasted if the victim, er, patient, wiggled around even a hair while the protons were being pumped in via an exacting software program. Even a millimeter off is fairly "off" when margin between full tissue blast and a mild suntan is measured in a couple of millimeters. So, nothing left to chance, a good securing was provided, my head and shoulders literally bolted to the treatment table courtesy of a breathable, hard plastic mesh apparatus custom-made for me. Descriptions of this accoutrement, now decorating a shelf in our den (and sporting a nifty fedora, tipped slightly down and left for effect) have run from "it's Hannibal Lecter's naptime!" to a torture device from a medieval fencing school.

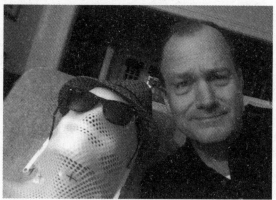

My Mask and me.

In this setup, my head and neck, encapsulated as they were in the funky mask and pinned tightly down, had really no chance of moving. My breath was not constrained at the rib cage, but certainly felt claustrophobically so at my mouth and nose, breathing through the holes in the mesh. I had a little taste of the problem during the almost comically weird mask-making; this involved a not-quite-piping hot sheet of perforated, flexible plastic, pulled out of what I could swear was a repurposed pizza-oven, and lain across my head, neck and shoulders. The ritual proceeded with assurances that no dermatologic disasters would be resulting. Then techs quickly smushed the heated sheet to conform to every contour of my balding pate, rugged jaw and bulbous Slavic schnozz, over shoulders and just north of nipples.[32] Then "hold still—it's got to harden, about twenty minutes." Another meditative moment!

I naturally fall into a meditative posture and routine when faced with a need or desire for stillness; I even practiced a little the weekend before treatment, meditating while lying flat as opposed to the usual cross-legged style. But I hadn't fully anticipated the tactile distraction of my mouth and nose utterly encased in plastic, however breathable it was.

So, to my heartbeat I moved again for an anchor. During the actual treatments, I must admit there was an interior battle to shift observation to my tumor itself as it was being ray-gunned. But that ginned up too much chatter and anxious tone—would it feel gone? Atomized? An angry ember? It was a bit distracting. Resting[33] back in my heart region was familiar and open. As some advanced practices (more on those later) center on sitting, or lying, with gratitude, that worked fine for me. Gratitude of having the good fortune of access to this truly bizarre but possibly life-saving event joined me with each beat.

Be the (TWA) Pilot

Whichever of these elementary practices that you take up, it can be helpful to cap the session with some relaxing of attention away from

---

32   Can the author comment on his nipples? Oh, yes, he can.
33   I just mistyped "roasting"...true, dat.

the specific target and just "open out," without an object, to whatever results. Just let the mind be for a little bit. See what happens and witness your awareness itself as it settles.

There's a quiet but important aspect of this seemingly "foot off the gas" move, and it's about that "meta" aspect of awareness—the faculty of the watching and its own varying qualities. When we release the intention from whatever wavicle of attention the day's practice was or turned out to be, it's natural to become a bit more aware of awareness itself—field and watcher in interaction. Getting to know the breath, the heartbeat, the body (and upcoming...the feeling state, the thoughts)—all are important. But a little regular practice of dropping the investigation and instead observing the quality of the watching itself helps uncover a felt sense of the whole, of unity.

There's a snippet from an old Buddhist prayer that captures this aspect of practice well:

> *"Don't look at what arises: be what knows the arising*
> *Like an oak stake in hard ground*
> *Stand firm in awareness that knows..."*

This may become the whole of the practice, sitting in the pilot's seat, even as pilot and airspace ultimately become perceived as all one big, "vibe-y" thing. Or not. But we can start early here in a routinized way to throttle back to a state of "landscape" mode, rest...and meta.

That Pivotal Moment

There is a recurrent moment[34] in which attention goes from present to not, and another from lost to, "Oh yeah, where was I?" I think this is a powerful two-step, not to be just tolerated or slogged through. Obviously, becoming more aware of attention slipping like Jell-O off

---

34   An understatement!

the spoon, and saving it from the gobbling dog[35] under the table is a useful skill in its own right. There is also value to be gained in what else may be discovered around these inevitable losses. The murderers of stable attention are legion. But most of us have just a couple of frequent offenders to become acquainted with.

Let's take a sample scene. You are humming along in the two-act practice, easily staying on the arc up to top of the breath, then down, then the body snapshot, and so on. At some point, another wavicle intrudes, or a mess of them do, and pull attention away. That event generates a particular, felt shift—energy of attention diverted into chasing the chatter, even adding to it. The shift, however subtle, can be identified and understood, just like a pulled muscle or a scratchy throat. We have to look closely to observe the monkey-mind as it dangles a banana and then swings away. A quantum speculation is that the energy of defending and chasing the new stuff in the field ultimately dissipates, leaving clear attention to reemerge.

At the other end of the energy spectrum, one can be similarly cruising when attention disappears into a tunnel before you ever get to switch the hi-beams on. That felt sense of a de-powering of mind can become familiar during and after, but harder to anticipate just before. How stable attention degrades into lost attention can be cryptic—what's happening just before the lights go out, what phenomena of mind are on stage just before the curtain drops without warning. That moment of return from distraction, I think, is even more opaque—like waking up or coming out of a reverie. What brings the mind back online? What leads the puppy back to the paper?

Yet with practice, attributes of "I'm slipping" become gradually more attuned to as you repeat the "tuned in...uh-oh" (out)...oh, ok, back aware" sequence again and again. Over time, we can pick up a felt sense of the sliding toward a loss of attention and the pivot back.

---

35   Gus loved Jell-O.

If clear attention is the base state, and our link to a deeper Vibe of belonging, then inattention is a coverup, a smudge on the camera lens. And where there's a coverup, there's usually fear—a fear of dropping into hard-to-hold suffering as an extreme example. Attentional losses are also what can generate critical self-judgment upon recognizing that pivot. That can be its own quicksand, right there, and what Dr. Kabat-Zinn nods to aspirationally in his adjective "nonjudgmental."

Instead of a crime, better to consider the event as a curiosity, even worth turning focus directly into. We just get back at it, as best as we can with the state of attention of our particular moment.

A fruitful tactic of seasoned meditators to attend to the loss of attention, whether of the "blizzard" or "tune out" type or anywhere in between, is to resettle and open to physical and emotional experience. These Three-Point and Two-Act practices help build some skill here. With practice, some ability to watch the loss coming and adjust a little—resettle and drop into the body and heart—develops and informs.

For Instance (A Report from Right Now)

This morning in my writing time, I anticipated my alarm prompt to meditate. I've been excited about practicing these core techniques as I write about them. I'm in an activated, pretty upbeat mood this morning, having received some positive medical news. Last night, the good news of an MRI report showing no new growth in the smallish, misbehaving protein in my cervical spine had me relieved, yet activated. I slept a little restlessly, my mind having some trouble downshifting from the last couple of weeks of uncomfortable tension.

So, plopping onto Pac-Man this morning, I hit my timer, wheezed my HWG, and started. A couple of minutes passed, I think, of solid attention to the breath, despite some nibbling thoughts about how to better frame this "pivot" issue in returning to my writing.

Then, a blizzard of ideas came...a graphic to help illustrate contracted attention on the breath. A camera lens? An eyeball of varying size? I need a cartoon mascot! Call it, hmmmm... Wavy the Wavicle! What would Wavy look like? Write it down!

Then...a stop and a pivot, a sweet recognition of being off on a wild ride into creative thought. It contrasted brightly with how my mind has been cooking with some anxious narrative over the last few days.

I settled, wiggled my ass briefly into my cushion as I "dropped into the body" to anchor myself—noting briefly a residual heaviness in my gut, but some edgy energy in my chest. By reflex, I reengaged the practice with a quick, rote H-W-G.

Act I, full, Act II, restless body. This went on for a half-minute or so, then, more hijacking thought—I should literally write about this gaining and losing attention that's occurring to me right now, as a useful, "meditator-on-the-street" example! Oh, that's great! It's so meta! Isn't it ironic that I'm not meditating while juiced about writing about the loss of attention? And I can write about that, too, and...oh.

This next pivot back to awareness of thought intrusion brought with it a brief judgment of "you poseur...how can you write about this stuff when you can't even f***king keep your attention on the breath to prove it to yourself?" It's a common judgmental narrative for me, an oldie but goodie, like hearing "Brandy, She's a Fine Girl," but with tubas and kazoos.[36]

I tossed off that minor, familiar self-trashing with a smile—"oh, that again." As an aside, that's taken some years of work to diminish—but that's just me.

---

36   Still would make my toe tap!

And...wiggle and feel my body, my heart, and off again. I struggled through the rest of the sitting, yet with some compassion, recognizing and accepting my mind would be tugging to get back at the keyboard but my intention was to be right here and now, just watching the breath.

Last week, my sessions were dominated by other, also familiar distractors. A couple of days went, "breathe...breathe...breathe...go dark." For me, dread commonly generates the defense of a blanket over attention, the tune-out side of things predominating over the monkey-mind described above. I had little control or anticipatory cues heading into the tunnel. But upon that sweet regaining of awareness, a practiced dropping into the body and heart yielded me some clarity about heaviness, medical worry, and a decision to shift the object of my attention to the worry itself—"turning into" the wavicle as best I could and sitting with what was really operating and causing suffering in me. Tough stuff, but that's adaptation in action.

Where This Fits In: Nailing the Basics Down

Some may be chomping at the bit at this point to move to the next set of practices. I've hopefully whetted your appetite for developing an expansive ability to observe the field, and then move to witnessing one's own patterning and defending—events kicking up feelings and thoughts, and then secondary judgment of that stuff. The more speculative but perhaps grander-sounding payoff of being able to hold onto that and sense the "Vibe" of belonging may also loom large and be enticing.

But please do not skimp on this basic set of practices. Stick with it and watch for a gradual improvement in your attentional skill set before moving on. Rushing through to gain a fragile pseudo-mastery in the core, elemental skill of attending, losing attention, and regaining it will inevitably lead to more struggle down the path.

Lesson time: my own initial attempt to learn to ski took place well into my forties. Shamed by my decent but certainly not SportsCenter-worthy rips down the "bunny hill" at a ski area at Lake Tahoe—that is, me and a humiliating gaggle of elementary school kids—I pronounced myself fit for a new color of "diamond" and risk. Bad idea, I learned shortly after getting off the lift way up the mountain. The ghoulish names of the runs should have been a clue.

You won't break your leg (nor did I) if you don't get comfortable and semi-competent with the basics of awareness practice using the breath. But the chances of losing faith in the practice when thought blizzards come, and complex pattern sets too, are a lot higher if you don't put in the early work.

How long does that take? Uncertainty prevails, but well, you'll sorta know it. Most folks who start off and expand their sitting to fifteen to twenty minutes per day notice some increased stability and clarity within about four weeks. But again, that month, or any, will likely be punctuated by days of "wow" and days of "this is impossible." Nevertheless, the general trend will be of gaining skill in directing, holding and regaining attention. But practice and experience are key.

Summing Up: Some Variations and the Pivot

We edged into the shallow end of the pool with some variations on basic breath practice and an alternative target—the heartbeat. Then we focused on that particular drama of losing and regaining attention. So, let us reinforce before we move on:

- 💬 We worked with a couple of ways of attending to the breath: a *simple observation, as an in/out/snapshot of the whole body (the "trey")* and as *a more fluid observation* of gathering air, releasing it, and with that release, an expansion of attention out to the whole body.

- We worked with another notable sensation of the body: the *heartbeat* as a target for awareness. I do encourage sticking with one anchor or style for at least a couple sessions unless it's really obvious it's doesn't work. "Switching horses" frequently, mid-stream, this early on in training, tends to be a sign of tension and even desperation in starting up this practice. It's better to use that struggle to build your ability to adapt.

- Speaking of attentional struggle, we looked at it directly with an emphasis on not shaming yourself off the cushion. Instead, approach the loss and regaining of attention, *the "pivot,"* as its own important thing to be curious rather than judgmental about. There are times that the particular "pivot" is present and recurrent enough to switch to it as the entity to observe. In any of these variations on the pivot and how to respond, *settle into a felt sense of the body and heart*, "drop into it" so to speak, in managing the state of the moment.

- Lastly, I was a nudge about letting the cement dry a bit on *some consistent sense of skill with watching the breath* before jumping the next set of practices. It will pay off as things get more complex.

Later, we'll walk out from a fraction of the physical sense of self, the breath practice, to exercises engaging a fuller awareness of the physical, emotional, and thinking aspects of self. That's our introductory map, that first cataloguing of mind. But before that, I want to give you an alternative map of the territory. We'll consider "operating systems"—a developmental, processing approach. As we'll see, the wave/matter seesaw is quite likely built right into the evolving brain.

PART II

CHAPTER 7

Another Map: Your Mind, the Operating System(s)

Hey, But We Got a Map Already

I promised you another "map"—an alternative framework to help guide what appears in the daily mindscape in meditation and in the rest of the day as well. This second map is a variation, based a different way to look at our experience—via the functional development of the brain. Why another approach? I've got some reasons.

One is linking subjective, interior, hard-to-measure meditating to some commonly known brain structures and functions helps us understand how change happens with practice: change in outlook, coping, and in adaptation to life has its correlates in neurology (and cardiology...stay tuned).

Another reason is wonkier. Forgive me as I wax nerdy about the elegance of a functional "operating system" (OS) metaphor for the evolutionary development of our brain function. In my clinical practice, it is useful for shrink and patient alike in explaining, say, how our limbic emotion can dent in a rational response in a conflict, or how our basic lizard-brain threat can overtake both of those. That those three are gradually being integrated and orchestrated by the next operating system, currently under evolutionary construction, is not only a thrilling prospect. It also supports this practice, as meditation is a particularly effective way to develop that newest aspect of the mind.

One more reason: it helps tie together the "parallel awareness" reality, that we each "construct" a separate, "little-m" self in our daily awareness but also are immersed in a broader, "big-M" field of energy. That very duality is reflected in brain structures and processes, especially in the layouts of aspects of the cortex and of two distinct attentional pathways that course through every brain—one that privileges separate self-awareness and the other an always-on attention capacity tuned to the broader field.

Mindfulness practices not only offer us the opportunity to know better the details of our individual "homes" of experiences and reactions, but also to access deeper levels of awareness, of that big-M field of belonging and connection that we'll explore in more detail in Part III. This alternative, functional map will help us understand what we observe in both of these realms.

The Mind, OS Style

This map of functional "operating systems," each one building on its prior iteration, was developed by the physician/researcher Karl Pribram and written about extensively by the child development expert Joseph Chilton Pearce and others. It frames four developmental levels of evolving brain, each with its correlative anatomy that has developed to meet the evolving challenges of humanity. Each OS represents a quantum (hah!) leap toward a higher, broader level of interaction in the big-M: from blunt survival of self, to interaction/connection/relationship, to ideas and creativity (generating new wavicles!), to integration and deeper connection with the big-M.

These OSs are not separate systems. As one of the contemporary bigshots of integrative philosophy, Ken Wilber, has observed, levels of organization don't leave the prior levels behind but rather they "transcend and include"—that is, preserve the functional goodness of the prior one and envelop it in the next novel, advanced design.

Here are the broad categories of your brain network:

1.0: Survival brain is the most primal, archaic OS, preserving the self by generating black-and-white, blunt signals of "win/lose" interaction—intense somatic phenomena—directed fear, panic anxiety, libidinous urges and pleasure, rage, deep depressive emptiness. It is mostly located in the brain stem and cauliflower-like cerebellum.

2.0: Relational brain is the neural complex one step up from threat and survival—correlating with the awareness of a relationship or interaction with another by generating the emotions of joy, longing, sadness, satisfaction, anger, and uncertainty that emanate from coexistent interaction with other wavicles in the field.

3.0: Idea brain, what most folks identify as "the" brain," is home to most of memory, symbolic thinking, analysis, imagination, and creative thought. 3.0 is a huge developmental advancement in the individual's interaction with the cosmos: toward creative acts contributing to the field, not simply apprehending and interpreting but actually generating new phenomena— innovation in all its lovely forms.

4.0 (currently under development): The integrative/ meta-aware brain representing the developmental next correlate—a set of networked connections located in the pre-frontal cortex, reaching out and tying into the other OS's and some other surprising places.

Eons of evolutionary development have grown a network of connections: survival brain talks to relational brain talks to creative/analytic brain, and back and forth to each other, like your gaggle of aunts after they heard you dented the car. We'll focus more deeply on these functional constructs, focusing on the phenomena each generates for our observation—including the newest, most exciting, but less figured-out addition to the home, busily gathering permits and tussling with the contractor.

OS 1.0: Slither Up

Let's imagine a little about how we went from utterly non-aware creatures to barely yet alarmingly aware creatures.

Picture yourself for a moment as a lizard—not thinking about the beauty of the jungle around you or how to best prepare the fly you've just captured as part of a reptilian tasting menu.

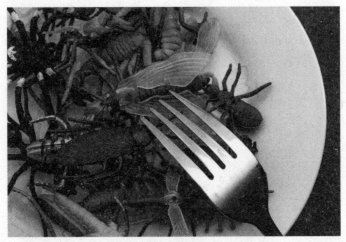

Pairs well with a Clos de Gecko.

No, you're just eating to survive, while your trigger-happy 1.0 stays lit up, vigilant for any other critter who's aiming to gobble you up while you're not paying life-or-death attention.

1.0 is the survival OS, anchored in the most basic, "I win/you lose" part of brain. The phrase "fight/flight" often is used to describe this OS; a fuller description includes "freeze," as in, "play dead." All three are basic threat responses to a "not-self," not rooted in coexistent interaction.

This is not the, "Does she like me?" part of brain, or the "Do these pants make me look fat?" part, which assume a more evolved quality of self-relating-to-another-self. (That's 2.0, coming up next.) It's the OS we got from our reptilian genetic friends, and sometimes may notice pops up in Uncle Louie at Thanksgiving dinner. While it sounds like a rather low bar in a broad cosmic sense, remember that even the most primal awareness represents a great evolutionary step beyond mere animate existence without any reflective awareness (fuzz atop the surface of sour cream in the back of the fridge/Uncle Louie after a six-pack).

1.0 is by nature a loudmouth of an OS, with physical, emotional, and mental/thought signals that are more local and intense. After all, in evolutionary history, 1.0 was once the only primordial signal system, operating for the goal of living to see another day and not caring much for style points.

Each of the "big three" states of suffering—"anxious," "angry," and "sad"—have a particular, more intense and primal feel when they originate from 1.0. A punch to the side of the head, a Dear John letter to the heart, or even a question on the quantum physics final that didn't seem to be covered in the professor's lecture (Heisenberg would suggest guessing "B," probably) can each generate a blinding 1.0 light on the dashboard of consciousness.

1.0 signals are sometimes so overwhelming and intolerable as to stun or freeze us from accessing higher centers of mind, and even co-opting the survival purpose. Here's an example, involving anxiety. My lovely wife, toddler son, and I were moving into our first home, which had been outfitted for the prior, elder owner with bright red, cold-war cliché medical alarm system buttons throughout. We'd ignored the "Mr. President, you may make Vladivostok an ashtray" triggers as we went about toddler-proofing the place. Alas, my industrious little man did not, hiking himself up on a chest full of blankets and sending Mother Russia a clear message.

The ear-bleeding alarm stunned his two addled parents, our quick trip to OS 1.0 momentarily disorienting us from recalling where we'd left the disarm codes and phone numbers. A pounding at the front door was ignored, then eventually registered; I opened the door to find a burly fireman winding up his axe like Paul Bunyan to take a whack. (More 1.0!) Ultimately higher brain centers snapped online.

We can define "anger" as the dashboard light of grievance among wavicles, with a spectrum of variation from getting frustrated by heavy traffic or the voice of the annoying guy in the next cubicle over, to the primal rage that can be generated by being messed with in a major-league, traumatic way. That 1.0 kind of anger is different, more cataclysmic. Similarly, 1.0 sadness feels different than garden-variety blues. Many individuals with the most severe impairments in temperament find the root of their pain here—a gruesome sense of early aloneness and alienation, of being left to fend for themselves.

Early-and-often childhood exposure to anxious "watch out," to grievous "not fair," and to depressive, "left and all alone" experiences can groove in an ongoing defensive posture and to deep difficulty in teasing out 1.0 vs. 2.0 or higher responses to later challenges. A contemporary "peacetime" life nevertheless still feels like a chronic risk of "wartime."

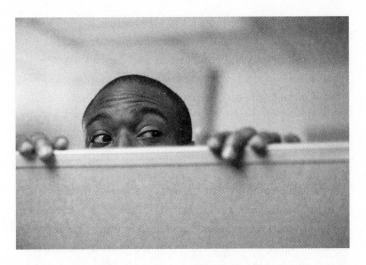

No, Todd, I haven't seen your latest cute cat video—by all
means, tell me about it!

1.0 can also become an all-too-familiar landing spot for other states
of suffering to collapse to—those experiences themselves generating a
fear that they are too hard to hold or adapt to. A catchphrase for this
I use with patients is "collapse to 1.0"—states of suffering that trigger
their own deeper survival fear. Mindfulness practices can be essential
in helping patients tease out the core "ouch" from the reactive
"OMG" and modify down that additional intensity. With practice,
adaptation develops of having held that hot potato before and made
it through.

2.0: Emo Brain

We've fortunately built upon the 1.0 "to be or not to be (eaten)"
OS to attend to the next great developmental wave in conscious
existence, heralded by the pithy question uttered by sweater-vest-
appareled therapists the world over:

"Do you have your copayment?"

I deeply apologize for that clinical compulsion. I actually meant:

"How do you feel about that?"

OS 2.0, the relational brain, is a complex web of connections—
hooking up "lower" and "higher" parts of the brain in a way that
echoes the greater purpose of attending to, yes, relationship. While
1.0 sits in the simpler "me vs. not-me," 2.0 manages our "me"
coexistence with other wavicles, with "not-me's" in their many forms.

Neuroanatomy texts refer to OS 2.0 as the "limbic" system. "Limbic"
means "border," as in the border between the reptilian/sensory 1.0
brain and the big fluffy 3.0 "thinky" cortex. It links ancient sensation
to pretty much all the other aspects of the brain. It's a complicated
network, akin to the dreaded jungle of wires behind your computer
desk or home theater.

The relational 2.0 has a couple of its own functional hotspots of note.
One is the amygdala, which I am required by tedious academic writer
statute to note is "almond-shaped," leading to much mirth in the
inevitable comedy lines linking "mind" and "nuts."

The amygdala serves a vital functional purpose in 2.0, linking what I
shorthand as the "video"—the sensory apprehension of an event—to
the first, rough reaction or judgment of that event, or what I'll call
the "soundtrack." The amygdala links up immediate apprehension of
experience to a first pass at, "How do I feel about it?"

Early in evolutionary development, the 2.0 system was heavy on
the soundtrack. There was just not as much for the early human to
know, learn, and retrieve intellectually. We can take for granted that
our own tremendous facility of memory and analysis (that's OS 3.0),
encoding the video, soundtrack, and color commentary of events,
has always been there as we experience it today. But early on, critters

leaned on 1.0 sensation for want of any other input. Those lizards with the primal neural flash of, "I shouldn't eat that bug, Harry keeled over just yesterday when he ate that," advanced their brand. (And Harry was delicious.)

So, what do we do with that video/soundtrack package? Let's consider another piece of 2.0 real estate, the hippocampus. It's also named for its shape: "*hippos-*" means "horse" and, weirdly, "*kampos-*" refers to a sea monster. So, yeah, "horsey sea monster." Let's go with "seahorse-shaped."

The location of this aquatic equine—bumping up next to the amygdala, and then winding around toward OS 3.0 cortical structures—hints at its utility. Hippocampus processes and filters those video/soundtrack packets of mind events and delivers them to 3.0 cortex and elsewhere. The hippocampus modifies the immediate imprint of events from the amygdala—call it a "file open on the desktop"—and holds it as a short-term memory file, ready to be stored or reinforced as a signal, or not, in the 3.0 cortex.

There is surely more to 2.0 than a nut, a seahorse, and a mess of wires. But the takeaway is that 2.0 takes our observation of events beyond mere experience and sensation to relationship and judgment. One (nutty) part of 2.0 attaches meaning to the experience, another (horsey, fishy) part prepares it for use in the next big leap in mind—the facility of thought in its rainbow of forms and types, 2.0 heralds the birth of emotion, an essential set of signals of our interactions in the "field." It's a step up into a *qualitative* form of experience, from a basic wail of a hungry infant or that same cutie's blissful look of bonding with Mom, to a highly refined signal system to inform our experience of events both trivial and profound.

The 2.0 emotional soundtrack develops in early life and can be tragically stunted and beaten up by early life trauma, too. Yet with mindfulness practices, it can also be entrained and cultivated as an essential tool through our lives.

3.0 Brain: Eureka!

"Eureka!" is an expression famously attributed to the Greek mathematician/physicist/all-round smart guy Archimedes (and to a prospector's eruption at stumbling over a gold nugget in 1850s California). Let's work with the first one in elaborating on the glory that is OS 3.0, also referred to as the "neocortex" or just cortex—the idea OS.

According to legend, Ol' Archie[37] was apparently primping for a toga party and, as he lowered himself in the bathtub for a soak, likely noticed for the umpteenth time that the water level rose along the sides of the tub as his stinky self sank into the water. We can walk through his sequential reactions.

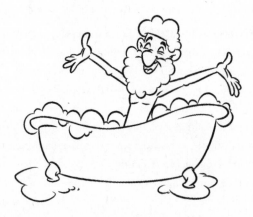

Archimedes' discovery of the Greek swear word "oipho." Look it up.

---

37   Probably not his real nickname.

His 1.0 brain would have registered safety, or perhaps a message of recoil at the temperature being too hot or cold.

Quickly passing the 1.0 "friend or foe" test, his 2.0 brain would have gone off with pleasure at the comfort of the water, or some displeasure at the lack thereof. His OS 2.0 registered a basic felt judgment of the experience—his relationship with the wavicles of water, of an observed change in the meniscus of the water in the tub,[38] and perhaps the lint in his filthy, filthy navel.[39]

Then, briskly to 3.0: his observation of the water level change triggered associations with other ideas he'd been working on involving displacement of a volume in fluid. A new "wavicle" idea about displacement and volume was given birth, right there in the tub. Via OS 3.0, new phenomena emerge into the great quantum soup of big-M, new wavicles for the rest of us to behold and interact with.

Archimedes's joyous reaction to what he'd just figured out, "Eureka!," is yet another bit of 2.0. History suggests he was so excited by his brainstorm that he sprang from the tub and ran down the street in his birthday suit, which I imagine generated still other 2.0 judgments from neighbors.[40]

Cortex, the sea-sponge-looking locale of OS 3.0, does so much we take for granted that we can forget its standard features were once luxury options on earlier models. Behold the bounty: cortex registers, organizes, and analyzes all sensory perception, and it issues movement (motor) commands. It takes inputs from experiences and works in both conscious awareness and subconscious "percolation," to guide our operations out into the field of big-M Mind. That sounds pithy, but it is a breathtaking evolutionary development. It seems obvious,

---

38   Wavicle doula (a Greek term, actually) was not available.

39   "Archimedes' Filthy Navel"—now an artisan cocktail in Brooklyn.

40   And "No toga, no thongs, no service" signs at early Grecian eateries.

but try getting your pet iguana (mired in 1.0, right?) to, say, play cards with you.

From 3.0, we not only note wavicle critters in our awareness, but also develop not only ideas about them but symbols in sound and sight—written and spoken language—from which we can share our experience of these new wavicles.

Whole libraries of texts have been written about the layout of structure and function in the cortex. The most basic involves the outer "gray matter" layer of microchips and hard drives, and the inner "wiring" of white matter. Another speculates on the divergent functions of the left and right hemispheres of the cortex, a tussle stereotypically pitting reason in one corner of the ring versus emotion in another.

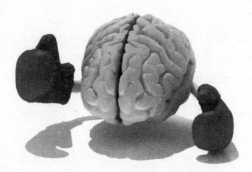

The battle of the hemispheres.

The left cortex, besides controlling the opposite, right side of the body in movement and sensation, has been associated with detail orientation, reason, and language. The right cortex, besides managing movement and sensation for our left sides, has been characterized as the creative, intuitive, artsy-fartsy part. Some archaic gender value judgments can flow from these generalizations. Spreadsheet Johnny is left-brained and has no skill set in divining why his wife is feeling verklempt at a sad movie; right-brainer artiste Judy is a melodramatic diva with little common sense. It's more complicated than that. Those interested in fuller detail are directed to the excellent writings of Dr. Iain McGilchrist, an English psychiatrist and author who has written deeply and well about the topic.

McGilchrist's work reinforces the map of functional brain development out of earlier OS's of mind (1.0 survival, 2.0 relational), then explains the lefts and rights of the 3.0 cortex (call them "3-L" and "3-R," perhaps) in a novel way in terms of function of awareness.

Left "brain"—left cortex, really, as there's no useful purpose in in categorizing a "left brain stem"—nails down *details*. McGilchrist really simplifies it to a single word: 3-L is the *"what"* cortex. It's for trees, not forest—a telephoto focus that maps the territory, cataloguing the wavicles in the landscape. Our series of interactions get organized into a series of "particle" snapshots.

On the other hand, McGilchrist emphasizes the *"open-field"* nature of right-brain awareness. 3-R is the *"how"* cortex, apprehending experience in context, process, and flow—a landscape function of our awareness to complement the telephoto function of the left brain. 3-R gives us open, spacious awareness associated with contemplative states (OS 4.0, as we'll cover coming up), but also survival-level vigilance against threat. Right brain immerses self-in-the-soup, tilting toward the "wave" (rather than particle) aspects of our experience.

The two hemispheres cross talk via a tough band of neural wiring called the corpus callosum (Latin for, um, "tough band"[41]) that connects the two. It manages signals between hemispheres, operating as a hall monitor.

To simplify, 3-L is more for details, 3-R for big pic. To me that's sensible, logical, beautiful—as we bloom out of survival, to

---

41   The Ramones mediating the hemispheres?

relationship, then to concept, we spring into a new form of mind(s) that can apprehend both the tight close-up and the vast panorama, the little-m mind of stuff and the big-M broader field.

OS 3.0 provides more complete tools to navigate reality, including our biggest advance, of idea creation. Thought is a whole new quantum wavicle. Prior to 3.0, wavicles bumped in a way that more or less just rearranged the wavicle deck chairs on the ship. 3.0 changed all that and changes it every moment in ginormous and tiny ways— for better, and sometimes worse. With every new discovery, from the wheel, to penicillin, to Velcro, to nuclear war, to that ditty you sung this morning in the shower, new wavicles come forth. We create and give to the cosmos, to the big-M, in this way.

4.0: What's New?

Underpinning this survey of the OSs of mind is a direction of development. So, what's new? What is the leading edge of the evolutionary development of mind? And where might that new OS be situated? For or all we know, we could be sitting on it.

What's new is an area of the brain right behind our eyes, termed the pre-frontal cortex—as in, the most forward part of the frontal cortex. Call it *"PFC."*

Look up "pre-frontal cortex" on the internet,[42] and you'll get some common terms that may suss out its role and function: "governor," "integrator," "galactic overlord." They all sound in the ballpark (except the last one), at least in terms of OS 4.0 observing the wavicle kitties[43] of the other OSs.

The evolutionary development of the OSs is actually mirrored in how they emerge in utero and infancy. Embryonic structures of all four

---

42 A rare use of the internet.
43 A less-rare use of the internet.

OSs are present in the first trimester of prenatal life, then develop in a sequential way at different paces. The PFC develops the most gradually—barely online as the third trimester progresses, and with maturing of structures, not really concluded until around baby's first birthday.

As with almonds, seahorses, and tough bands, we may sleuth out what 4.0 does by where's it's located and what it's plugged into. Found up and behind our eyes, the PFC is perfectly situated as a kind of über-conductor orchestrating the signals of the other OS layers—survivalist, relational, and rational. Express routes to brain stem, limbic, and cortex emanate from the PFC, suggesting it mix-masters the wide range of wavicle phenomena to produce our overall awareness. That's an incredibly important development—4.0's role as the meta-aware aspect of brain allowing us to integrate internal signals.

Recent functional imaging and other techniques reveal another surprising link from the PFC—to an extensive network of neural tissue in and around the heart. The heart! The heart's own neural network generates an electromagnetic field that is stronger than that of brain tissue. What's that for? There are also express routes to and from the GI tract, though those are not as extensive as at the cardiac ones. The purpose of these surprising links is not fully understood, but there is clear neuroanatomic evidence of a "conversation," with pathways heading northward from heart (and gut) to head to parallel those heading south.

While OS 4.0 serves to integrate "inward," it may also serve a broader next step in attention: to reach outward in awareness beyond the little-m self. That measurable electromagnetic signal actually pulses out from each of us with every heartbeat. It could be impactful— empathy as waveform—or maybe just symbolic. Yet studies examining the modification of that signal with meditation practices, opening to the whole field itself, are promising. For now, we can at least wonder about how ascertainment of self-in-the-vibe is registered in the wavicles called you and me. As unusual as its sounds, "love" and "quantum" may literally belong in the same discussion.

Attention, Please

The cortex features a couple of other pieces of real estate worthy of our, uh, attention. Our capacity to attend to experience in and with the landscape runs via a complementary pair of routes, with surprising, distinctive functions that reinforce the little-m/big-M duality of our reality.

It's a framework elaborated on by the neurologist, author, and seasoned Zen meditator to boot, Dr. James Austin, who has meticulously studied how, in neuroscience terms, meditative practices impact the brain. His encyclopedic *Zen and the Brain* and more recent *Meditating Selflessly* are fine examples of his work.

Austin nicknames the two pathways with titles that sound like yoga poses: "top-down" and "bottom-up." Each pathway accounts for a different kind of awareness. Yes, it's telephoto versus landscape mode again.

The "*top-down*," or "*dorsal*" path in anatomy-speak, is an over-the-top route from parietal lobes over your scalp into frontal lobe. This attentional path streams specific, voluntary, directed attention from a perceived observing self: I see a tree, I pick up an idea from a book, etc. Austin describes this attention as "egocentric"—not meant as narcissistic snark, but instead highlighting it as a "self" looking at a "not-self." It logs "*whats*"—particular features of the field attended to from the frame of reference of the observer, as opposed to a more global awareness. It's the telephoto aperture on our camera of awareness, attending to the specific entities that we apprehend and relate to from our individual vantage points.

The other "bottom-up" or "ventral" attentional path starts in the low, in-back occipital lobes and sweeps forward and up to our frontal lobe. It streams continuously, a background awareness of the whole landscape. Austin dubs this one "allocentric—referring to the "perspective of things as themselves." In our discussion of this for my own clarity, he informed me that this kind of attention is "chiefly *not* referring back to [each of] us." "Bottom-up" attention is our base state of awareness, the effortless, self-free awareness we popped out into the world in. It's always been there, but we commonly override it by habit with our voluntary "top-down" attention, reinforcing a constructed position of separation. Sound familiar?

Yet events and interactions boil endlessly and scream for our (top-down) attention—especially thoughts linked to a physical/emotional soundtrack. We tend to identify with these linkages as an aspect "self," as me—or at least as a new bauble to be mesmerized by, like shiny keys shaken in front of the baby. Meditation helps us train our "top-down" attention to see them as momentary events on the horizon of a field of broader, "bottom-up" awareness. That top-down attention training, the fruit of our practices in Parts I and II, also gives us the opportunity to uncover, recover, or perhaps discover in Part III the "bottom-up" attention path—the always-on sense of immersion, separate from the top-down specifics of "me and it" to just "this"...one endless ocean of big-M, always there.

Eureka (Redux)

We've sketched out a second map, an evolutionary/functional depiction of the operating systems of mind. With each successive OS, there is development taming the rougher edges of its predecessor OS and including it as a chassis for the next new features. Each successive stage represents an inevitable push toward more complexity and fulfillment. Eureka, indeed.

We've practiced with the introductory concepts and tactics of beginning meditation using the basic map. Now that we've got an alternative map based in evolutionary development and direction, let's move back to practice and some more complex ways to use mindfulness. Both maps will come in handy as we explore our own mindscapes going forward.

CHAPTER 8

Back to the Cushion: Body and Heart

Our next steps build on the skills in directing attention to a physical target—the breath, most likely, but perhaps the heartbeat also—and expand that to observe other aspects of the physical. This tool is itself a valuable asset in terms of basic stress management, as Jon Kabat-Zinn has popularized in MBSR (Mindfulness-Based Stress Reduction).

Body awareness also provides another opportunity to practice that "meta" skill of losing and regaining attention. Awareness of certain aspects of the physical self can often be a powerful, sometimes even traumatic, generator of other phenomena. Individuals often defend by hyper-focusing on or ignoring the body, and with lots of secondary judgment. So it's essential to master tuning in to the body—pinkie toes, kneecaps, the gut, the space between the shoulder blades, all of it. We'll use the punchline, "dropping into the body," as a kind of shorthand for deliberately redirecting attention south of the cranium, including coincident emotional/feeling states—the more local aspects present in the moment.

We'll cover a couple of spins on the "body" area of practice, starting with a preparatory tactic called progressive muscle relaxation, "PMR" for short. We'll advance to a more detailed body scan practice, then a shorter version, likely familiar to those who have done MBSR. We'll focus on the moving attention around, in this case from the breath to another aspect of the physical self, and back. The body and heart are often rich in targets for repetitive distraction—a particular area of the body or feeling state routinely driving pre-occupation or slippage into tune out. We'll work on a variation specifically about the senses, and another attending to states of physical suffering.

One last hall-monitor comment: some eager folks may want to jump forward regardless of sufficient mastery of breath awareness and "gain-lose-gain-repeat" attention work. That's your call. But if you struggle mightily in moving ahead, there need not be cranky judgment in going back to work on the basic ground strokes of meditating on the breath. It's not a race to the next practice; moreover, whole schools of meditation begin and end with working solely with the breath, with beneficial results. So use or perhaps suspend your judgment, as needed.

Let Me Feel Your Body Talk (Your Body Talk)[44]

Generally, a body part attended to leads to awareness of any discomfort inherent there, and to some combination of an active attempt to change the suffering and acceptance of adapting to what can't be changed about it. Just bringing attention to the suffering self/ part often brings some benefit.

Directed awareness at the physical self, part by part, is the center of this exercise. Most sequences take a geographic approach, like with the PMR exercise we'll review in a moment—picking one end of the body and attending to it, then incrementally moving upward or downward. One may take the time and precision to include each toe tip, to the ball of the foot, to the arch, to the heel, up the lower

---

44   For you Olivia Newton-John fans. Leg warmers may come back "in style," eventually. Millennials, google it, or find the esoteric subreddit on it, or something.

leg, and so on. A very slow, deliberate, careful attempt to tend in awareness to each area of physical real estate is a useful practice all its own.

It's also useful to have in your bag of skills a truncated version. A short scan (lower body, abdomen, upper chest, head) can be built-in as part of an overall launch routine. I personally use a variation of this scan, right after "HWG," in grounding my awareness at the outset of a sitting. It's like running scales at the beginning of piano practice or doing some stretching before setting out on a run.

This is a good moment to reiterate the inevitability of losing attention during body/emotion practices. Wandering off into thought or fuzzing out is just as likely in this realm of meditation as any other, so no need get lit up about it. In fact, that "meta" angle is important here, as an eye out for what physical sensations/parts of the body/emotional states are likely to yank awareness out of clarity or stability.

Each of us have a lifetime of experience in memory, bonded in association to the physical/emotional "soundtrack" that was co-occurring with each experience, sometimes intensely so. The body "remembers." Physical awareness practices can be remarkably powerful in bringing implicit but repressed old memories and linked physical and emotional aspects into open awareness. A common early sign of such events can be the noting of one part of the body scan that either lights up tension or routinely drives awareness into a tunnel.

Waking Up to the Body

Actually locating the body parts to attend to can be difficult, whether in actively trying to relax muscles or to be more of a still observer of the felt state in a body scan meditation. It's not that unusual for many of us to "tune out" the body, especially its sufferings, and go "head first" in awareness, overvaluing our intellectual activity.

I think of Progressive Muscle Relaxation (PMR) as "poor man's biofeedback," a therapeutic technique that allows for an individual to gain control over a part or function of the body via a sensor to a device that provides evidence such as an alert or other information on a computer screen. PMR approximates the aspects of muscle biofeedback without the wires, computers, or super-villainesque associations to attaching an individual to electrodes. There's no rocket science here—just a routine of sequential flexing/tightening of a group of muscles briefly, then a releasing/relaxing of that group. It can be helpful to pair the exercise with some self-generated or recorded visualization cues, such as being on a beach, or in a luxurious spa tub, or whatever works for you; you may imagine the sun getting brighter in the sky, or the bath feeling more comfy as you sequentially relax yourself.

While the inevitable relaxing of muscle tension is undoubtedly a good thing, the secret sauce for me here is in engaging a practice of directing attention. As it's not a formal exercise in meditation, but a preparatory practice, I'm not calling it "No.1."

Body Exercise No. 0.5: PMR

Find a comfortable place to relax with all your muscles at gravity: lying on a bed, sitting in a chair with a high padded back for your head or lying on a carpeted floor will all do. Before starting, make a mental rating (one to ten) of how tense your muscles feel.

- **Start with your left hand. Clench it in a fist for a count of three, then release it slowly to a count of three.** Breathe deeply and slowly while you tighten and release. **Compare the feeling** in your left hand to your right hand; notice the difference.

- **Now tense your right hand for a count of four, then release** for a count of three. Remember to breathe deeply and slowly as you learned in the relaxation breathing exercise.

- Now move to your **forearms**, first tensing and releasing the left forearm (three count), then a pause to **compare the difference,** then repeat with the right forearm.

- Next, apply the same process to your **upper arms**—first left for a three count, then a pause, then the right. Keep **breathing deeply** and slowly.

- **Your shoulders and neck** are next. Shrug your shoulders (both sides at once) to a three count, and then relax. Work your neck by pressing your head back hard (1-2-3) and relax, then touch your chin to your chest (1-2-3) and relax.

- Your **face** is next (no mirrors for this part!) Wrinkle your forehead into a deep frown (three count) then relax. Close your eyes tightly (1-2-3) and relax. Grin as wide as you can and relax. Purse your lips tightly, then relax.

Next is your upper body. **Stretch your chest muscles** by taking a full breath, holding for three, the exhaling. **Arch your back** tightly (1-2-3); relax. **Suck your gut in** tightly (1-2-3), then relax.

- Next are the **hips and buttocks**. Tighten together (three count), then relax.

- Lastly, **work on your legs**—first thighs, then lower legs, then feet and toes. With each group, progress as you did with your arms: **tighten and relax** on the left, then **pause to note the difference**, and then do the same on the right.

Pause for a moment and note the difference in how your muscles feel, compared to your one to ten rating of your tension at the beginning of the exercise.

It's a good basic technique, helpful for easing the way into sleep at night, and on long car or plane trips. And it sneaks in some practice at directed awareness, too.

Body Practice No. 1: Toes to Head

This is a basic body scan exercise best done on your back or in a chair, rather than in a cross-legged position, which can challenge the body part "finding" below the waist. While it can certainly be done with eyes open, I've usually found closed eyes more helpful to reduce other stimuli and even to visualize the body area being attended to. But if eyes-closed leads to snoozy time, then go with eyes open.

- **Settle** into your usual position; set and start a timer if you choose; consider a **centering, starting routine** such as "Here-We-Go." In this case, the "Go" intention is ultimately moving attention to a sequential **scanning of the physical self.**

- Start with a **basic breath practice** to engage attention and reacquaint yourself with your awareness as a tool. Hold attention, lose it, bring it back, repeat.

- At a time of your choosing, **move** the focus of your attention to the **tips of the toes** of your left foot. Be aware of their felt sense—any sense of them touching, tingling, any pain, temperature, the feeling of them in your socks.

- **Repeat** that experiencing with the toes of your right foot. Feel all ten piggies.

- **If you lose attention, head back to the "home base"** of the basic breath practice. Resettle, then when you're ready, **move back** to your "Go" intention: the body.

- **Inch your awareness** northward to the balls of your feet—one then the other. Proceed with your arches, your heels. Notice the sensation of both feet together.

- **Advance** your attention to your **left lower leg**—skin sense, muscle tension, whatever you perceive. Repeat with the **right side.** Then to the knees, left and right, and the upper legs. Don't panic if you lose yourself in 3.0 thoughts, or tune out—**back to HWG, a few breaths, and then rejoin** your survey of your own territory.

- **Advance to your backside and pelvis.** Feel your butt, and your private parts, and your lower gut. It's ok if you become aware of uncomfortable distractions and attentional losses here and decide to make this step brief. These areas can sometimes be a challenge due to discomfort, or sometimes due to shame or trauma (more on this below). Note that, then move on when you're ready.

- Pull your view out to an **overall awareness of the lower half of your body.** Pause there, holding your entire lower half in attention. Feel it all, try to hold it all.

- A couple of breaths, then move your attention northward. **Attend to your abdominal area**—muscles in some degree of relaxation or tension, intestines at rest, burbling or making music. As before, it's no big deal if/when you **lose attention. When the "sweet spot" of becoming aware** you've gotten lost occurs, note it, hopefully without much judgment, and rejoin your survey.

- Advance upward to your **upper chest**. This should be more familiar; dwell a few moments on the quality of the **in and the out-breath**; notice the beat of the heartbeat; and take in the sense of tension of the **rib cage**, any heartburn, whatever is there.

- Follow around the rib cage to **the back and its layers of muscles**. Note how loosey-goosey or banjo-tight they are. You can follow out the experience of one shoulder and **slowly down the left arm**—upper arm, forearm, and to the sensitive hand with its palm, fingers, fingertips. Use your attention like a spotlight, following back up the arm to the middle spot between **the shoulder blades**—a very common repository of stress-related muscle tension. Repeat your slow examination tour of **the right shoulder and arm**, sequentially down to the fingertips and back.

- Back between the shoulder blades, take a moment to observe where the attention is settled, and **check back in with the cycle of breathing** for a few moments. Then, time to move north toward the finish.

- Move to your **neck and throat**—another common area of tension. Take a mindful swallow if it helps locate the experience.

- Move attention to your **head**, taking note of any tightness in face, scalp, and/or jaw. Note the inside of your mouth, how your tongue and teeth feel. Witness any pressure in your sinuses, behind and around your eyes.

- Turn your attention to the **inside of your skull**—does it feel light, heavy, in pain? This can be another tricky spot as a quick association to thoughts can lead to a loss of awareness of the basic experience of the inside of your head. You know what to do.

- Next, open the aperture out from the inside of your head to **take in the whole body**, include the whole survey just completed. No pressure to note every quark of detail or remember it all, just open to it as a practice in directed awareness. **Take stock of the entire physical you**—take a minute or two.

- Finally, **relax your attention completely**, letting it go where it wants. Pull back to the observer, that intermingling of self and field, and let it be. If you are so inclined, end with a "bookending" routine such as **"TWA"** or one of your own choice.

This is a fairly detailed, complete routine. But there's no need to get rigid about how to cover the territory. Starting at the head and working down, or starting at the fingertips and working in like in the PMR exercise, or a routine of your own concoction, all work fine. Find a sequence that suits you.

You may want to develop a "quickie" variation as part of a daily routine—a couple of breaths to tune into the lower body and legs, a couple for the torso and arms, a couple more for the head and neck—to bring the felt body "online." And on the other side of the spectrum, you can choose to train your attention on a particular nook or cranny. The added benefit in that practice, frankly, is less about "can I sense my spleen?" than in noting when and where attention veers away and gets lost, and practicing bringing it back. That trains the meta thing and can expose shadows and rabbit holes in awareness.

It's important to reinforce the comment I made above about body scans and potential, painful surprises. Re-experiencing of the memories of physical and especially sexual trauma can arrive in physical attentional practices. A focus on an aspect of 1.0 can generate powerful 3.0 (memories) and 2.0 (emotional reactivity). Both of those can feel catastrophic, risking a threat reaction, a collapse to 1.0. As with any work in mindfulness, using skillful means includes self-care. This does not preclude bodily practices for those wrestling with old wounds who could benefit from guidance from a therapist and/or meditation teacher.

Body Practice No. 2: The "Breathe Into" Tactic (Be a Balloon Dachshund)

This variation can become a truly useful way of practicing both body awareness and the facility of directing one's attention. It's true that our attention can be mostly in "landscape" mode, and thus aware of the "metronome" of our breathing in the background, but then concentrate our focus—telephoto-ing on the uvula, or the state of emotional feeling, or whatever the wavicle main target is. Remember back from the early chapter on neural pathways of awareness that we have "tracks" for each—with "open out" and the "close in" functions? This variation uses a little of both.

This covers the same physical ground of other body scan exercises but uses the anchor spot of the breath as a home base or gathering spot with each in-breath. We then "breath into" each of the areas of the body.

The variation:

- "Gather" and bring attention to the in-breath (wherever you choose to observe that in-breath

> from—chest, belly, nostrils, etc.). Then with the out-breath, direct awareness out to, say, the left foot;
>
> 💬 With the next in-breath, gather attention back, then "breathe it out" to, say, lower leg, and back to the in-breath at your anchor, and so on. Find a rhythm.

There's a quality of "breathing awareness into" each sequential piece of real estate, "inflating it" with your attention; then "gathering" the awareness back to your breath as anchor; then sending it out to the next spot. You can use the same sequencing as described above, or your own sequence, but with a rhythmic in-to-the-breath, then out-to-the-body swing.

Ultimately, as you complete the survey, you may...

> 💬 Finish with a sense of gathering up awareness on the in-breath, then expanding out to the whole of the body.
>
> 💬 End with just dropping any target and simply attending to the "bare" experience—and to the quality of the observing self. T-W-A.

It's sensible to work with this practice for at least a couple of weeks to get the hang of it and feel its benefit. That also allows for a certain awareness of what parts of the personal real estate may generate difficulty to become more aware of by their intensity or their resulting in a routine loss of stable attention. Like with basic breath practice, one can stick with this on an ongoing basis for great, sustainable benefit. Inevitably, the stressors that occur in pattern sets of reactivity will reveal themselves in body practice, there to be comprehended and adapted to.

Body Practice(s) No. 3: Open to Your Senses

Body scan practice can illuminate a split between "inner" directed phenomena—inner physical sensations like pain, muscle tension, heartbeat, and of course, the breath—and the five senses that gather data from the soup outside each of us. As a separate practice, it can be fruitful to tune into our senses (vision, hearing, taste, smell, touch), each a rich aspect of the field.

Working with the senses has its own rich history and many variations. In what is referred to as "ecstatic practice," attention is trained on a scene either large (like a grove of trees gently swaying in the wind) or small (a candle flame or a single flower bud in a vase). With some practice in simple, bare observation, it's not unusual to become more aware of details commonly passed over in everyday awareness, and to witness an increased vividness of color and form. Of course, sometimes it's mundane, and thus an ironic opportunity for meta practice: getting pulled into distraction, perhaps with thoughts of "just a dumb flower, I want to go take a nap," and the like, to work with as distractions to pivot back from.

Mindful movement practices mentioned earlier (Qi Gong, Tai Chi, yoga, walking meditation) are also forms of sense practice. The object of awareness is the experience of motion of the body, the touch of the feet on the ground. You can pick one sense and run (ok, maybe walk) with any as the objection of attention for your sitting or for movement. Alternatively, consider a tour of senses at one setting. Taking a rest break in the middle of a hike on a rock by the stream, one can practice this way:

> 🗨 Settle into a comfortable position; prep, a deep breath with each... Here: This unique place I am immersed in; We: Even here, aware of others working

(I'm just on a cool field trip!); Go: open out to a sense...or senses, one by one.

- Settle into a pattern of observation by letting the breath move to its natural state. If it's calm, note that. Still panting a little from that last hill, ok. Reengage the observing you with this simple practice.

- Take a quick "tune in" to your body as a whole by a quick scan. "Breathe into" it, so to speak, if you like that tactic.

- When you're ready, pivot to sense observation—one or a sequence. With any of these you may move breath awareness to the background or employ the "breathe into" variation of gathering awareness in the in-breath and releasing it to your specific attention to vision, hearing, smell, touch, etc. in the out-breath.

- If you're working with one sense, then attend to it. Let's start as an example here with your visual sense. If "framing" a whole scene, open in your visual awareness to that whole scene. Stay still and let the visual field of that view be your frame, like a painting.

- Keep the focus of attention on the visual. Watch how it may change in vividness or sharpness of color. Other senses, or emotional reactions, and/or thoughts are naturally going to arise in the midst of this practice; note them, "catch and release," and return to your visual observation intention.

- If the object in observation is a smaller-scale one, just stay with it (though it is certainly ok to move yourself to another point and practice from a different angle). Just attend in vision to the small

scene, mindful of the inevitability of other stuff
occurring, as mentioned above.

- Close the practice in your usual way: a move back
  briefly to the breath; then a letting go of any
  direction of awareness, just letting your mind be and
  resting back in the "watcher." There, we, are.

Be deliberate with each visual space, broad or intimate, in giving the
scene its full due. It's fine to move to another visual tableau—up at
the trees instead of down into the brook, for instance; but you're
working on attention, not trying to visually "snap every photo."

If you choose to work in a sequential way through more than one
sense, a brief shift back to the breath can separate each segment,
like so:

- Recenter on breath for a few beats, then pivot to
  a focus on the sounds all around you. Let yourself
  settle into the field as a "sonic" one, attending to the
  major noises and the subtle ones too, co-occurring.
  Rest in the observing of the whole orchestra, the
  entire auditory display.

- Recenter on the breath for a few moments, then
  turn your focus to the smells present. Rest in the
  observing, and "catch and release" if a particular
  sensory moment pulls attention away.

- After another return to breath watching, attend
  to the "touch" aspect of sense. Witness the tactile
  contact with what you are standing or sitting
  on. Feel the breeze on you. Note the sensory
  boundary between the self and not-self, which likely
  includes clothing. (Or not, if the practice is done in
  the shower.)

(Literally tasting the field might be a little dangerous, unless it involves something edible as the wavicle object of attention. More on that in a moment.)

💬 As with the single sense practice, close the practice in your usual way: a breath, then a letting go, resting back in the "watcher." There, we, are.

Variations on a Sensory Theme: Listen Closely, Smell the Roses

In working with one sense rather than working through all of them, pick a path down one of the five senses. With each, you can employ the basic attending or consider the variation of "breathing into" the sounds of the moment, or the taste, or the tactile sensation. Using the balloon-man "breathing into" tactic, breathing in to gather attention, breathing out into the sense to attend the experience, is a useful practice.

Let's take sound. Mindful listening allows for a deeper appreciation of the complexity of sound. It's a fruitful practice at the seashore or in a park or cityscape, with headphones attending to a piece of music, or in simply listening to the ambient, subtle variations in sound inside and outside an empty room in your house or office space. "Opening out" auditory attention to let it all in hones vital attention skills. Those auditory triggers that pull attention off into emotional reactivity or avoidance via thought-heavy narrative are also useful to know, by repetition and comprehension.

Working with olfactory (that's smelling) awareness is usually best done in a nature setting such as a park or flower garden; restaurants and food markets work well, too. Bringing attention to the quality, intensity, and change of scent as you sit or stroll can generate powerful associations and memories.

Practicing tactile awareness is a built-in aspect of the mindful movement work we referenced before but is also a reasonable thing to do in a safe uninterrupted setting. One can slowly and carefully engage simple touch awareness of the rock you are sitting on, the softness of the moss, the chill of dipping fingers in the stream. It can be a simple as the touch of the rug underneath and the clothes you are wearing. Without banishing this book to the back of the "erotica" section of the local bookstore, tactile practice on the various physical regions of one's loved one has its own rewards (but obviously poses its own interesting distractions).

Variations on a Sensory Theme: The Slow Food Movement

The same routine can be done with careful attention to the act of eating. This sense has been well-defined as deeply associative in awareness. Proust's description of an explosion of memory in a taste of a single French snack cake comes to mind; my grandma Sazima's chicken soup does, too.

The classic, even cliché, but effective and user-friendly exercise often done in MBSR classes involves the slow, incremental attentional eating of a single, humble raisin. It's actually not just an exercise in the taste sense, unless you mindlessly pop it in your maw and swallow. Try this instead:

- 🍇 Settle, HWG, and some settling breaths; then behold a single raisin between thumb and forefinger.
- 🍇 Observe it in vision: wrinkled, deeply colored. Can you see Millard Fillmore's face?
- 🍇 Feel it in your fingers: note the ridges, the give if you squeeze it a little (not too hard, now).

- Take a whiff of it (or perhaps in the box it came from)—ripe, grapey.

- Place it on your tongue, but no chewing yet—tongues work for touch as well as taste—note the shape, the crinkles, all of it.

- Take a chew. Note the gumminess, where it sticks. Roll it around your tongue, letting all of your taste buds have a survey before swallowing. Sweet, maybe tart, maybe you got a sour one.

- Then, swallow it. Try to attend to it, all the way down your gullet.

Obviously, this is a ridiculously slow, methodical process of eating a single raisin (or a cookie, or lasagna, or whatever).

Eating every single bite this way would be a diet plan likely ejected by Jenny Craig for its tedium. But as a way to notice all that is actually going on to attend to, it is a helpful tactic in weight control issues due to "mindless" oral gratification. Ramming a handful of fries down your fry-hole from the bag in the seat next to you without much awareness, that habit may change.

In a broader way, the practice reiterates how much we often mindlessly let go, whizzing by in the moment, a simple sensation: the ingestion of a raisin, or the first surprise of a raindrop on the cheek, or the beholding of a child's smiling face. Everything is an opportunity for some practice, in this way.

Body Practice No. 4: Working with Physical Suffering

One last body exercise is worth elaborating on: physical discomfort. Like with living in general, it's inevitable, and generates an opportunity to develop apprehension and comprehension of, and some adaptation to, the discomfort.

Concurrent, already-there physical suffering, whether aches and pains of the drop-in-acute or the simmering-in-the-background variety, are undeniably the norm rather than the exception for most of us, especially as we age. Aside from that built-in ache, the act of sitting in meditation almost always can generate some discomfort. Tight legs, numb feet, and sore back muscles are the biggies. Lastly, somatic discomfort can sometimes manifest as an aspect of practice— phenomena occurring during practice that can serve to distract or inform.

What to do? Well, one thing not to do is to play-act like the suffering is not there. All phenomena in the field of the moment are valid and worth attending to, so deniers beware.

A brief body scan at the beginning of any sitting is helpful to know what coexisting, perhaps competing somatic wavicles are present right from the get-go. "Meditating today with a sore neck" is a common catch-and-release moment for me as I proceed into my practice on any given morning.

While there may be concurrent discomfort from the outset of a sitting, there are also the events of a wavicle of physical suffering arising during the sitting. My advice applies to both: treat the wavicle kindly, like a squalling toddler at a restaurant. Ignoring or even screaming at the little one generally yields poor results, as any decent parent knows or learns. I have some options to offer based on the intensity of the tantruming wavicle of back pain, or leg spasm, or whatever.

At the very least, if the suffering is mild but present and distracting you from your intended awareness practice, "give it a seat nearby," akin to sitting your kid down within smiling distance, perhaps with an occupying toy. (With our three boys, neither my wife nor

I traveled without an EHW—"Emergency Hot Wheel"—in the pocket. Oddly, none of our sons are now on the NASCAR circuit.) Note the suffering sensation briefly as you would a passing thought, giving it a little attention, then return to your intention as the main event. If the suffering occasionally intrudes, turn briefly to it and witness it, even breathe into it as we've discussed, then back to the plan. It's what you got today, and that's ok.

If the suffering in more intense, more "code yellow" in terms of intruding on your intended practice, well, the toddler metaphor here changes to "sit on your lap and jiggle."

The intention changes to "there that's painful wavicle and my other intention"—watching them both, together. It's not easy, but not impossible, either. As your well-laid plan to focus on three-point breath practice is intruded upon by some persistent and distracting shoulder pain, grievance or disappointment may well arise, as can pity or self-criticism. It's all worth observing, or trying to.

If the squalling wavicle is truly overcoming your efforts to hold to the plan, you likely need to, as they say in football, "call an audible" and attend fully to your squalling kiddo. One can "turn into" the pain— attending specifically to the experience fully, switching it specifically to the object of your attention. Focusing on it in bare awareness or via "breathing into" it, you may experience its ebbs and flows of intensity, and what emotional tones the sensation may cogenerate—grievance, helpless sadness, anxiety, or dread—even some gratitude if a certain physical tension eases to relief. The painful sensory wavicle can be a signal leading to understanding and resolution or adaptation. Sometimes some directed attention into the suffering, some calming of it, can then allow for a return to the prior scheduled programming.

One other option needs noting for reasons of compassion and common sense: sometimes if it hurts too much to continue, then just stop and call it done for now. Pay the bill and take your little one to the park or back home for a nap. You can take a break and if in better shape afterward, try to come back to sitting with "HWG" and the prior intention or check back in with the suffering. You may try to shift into a walking meditation that allows for holding the pain better.

Or call it a day and get up. This is healthy training in coping, not the Spanish Inquisition. (No one expects that advice.)

Summary: Stay in Touch

We've covered a span of approaches to getting in better self-aware touch with your physical wavicles. From a preparatory self-care practice of PMR, we walked through a thorough and quickie body survey and some individualized breakout practices for the individual senses. We finished with some particular approaches to a painful but incredibly common act of sitting with physical suffering. I've suggested strongly that you incorporate them into a kind of regular sequence of:

- 💬 an introductory tune in (such as "HWG")
- 💬 anchoring via your most practiced aspect (breath watching)
- 💬 pivoting to the "Go" intention of your choosing (in this case, some aspect of witnessing physical phenomena); a bare witnessing of the physical phenomena, or a more rhythmic, swinging "breathing into" the target are both effective
- 💬 humbly anticipating the inevitable losses of attention during any practice and keeping a little eye out for which "trigger" wavicles may repetitively cause losses of attention
- 💬 closing the practice with a letting go of effort, resting back in the watcher with an eye out for what happens to attention, and then a closing routine ("TWA")

As I alluded to at the beginning of the chapter, "dropping into" the body and heart generally works best as a couple—an observation of the physical sense of self and the associated "weather" of observed emotional tone that co-occupies the moment. Practices on this are up next, along with a way of marrying them in one "dropping in" survey using an ancient map.

CHAPTER 9

Emotions Practices: Just Dropping In

Let's turn to awareness of the emotional tone of self.
Emotional or "feeling" states are conceptual names we use to describe a pastiche of the physical and mental. We all can identify with the labels for common emotional experiences: sadness, "peak" joy/ecstasy, anger, (directed) fear, "simmering" anxiety without a clear trigger, happiness/contentment, and the tension of uncertainty. We can even identify the "meh" of neutrality or boredom.

Each of us has a particular experience for these as individual as a fingerprint. It's good training to examine our own states and to know them well. The core knowing is mostly physical; secondary reactions manifesting in other realms—physical, rational, and awareness—may also be present. The whole schmear—the "pattern set"—is important to understand better.

Unfortunately, these emotional felt states in meditation are also prone to triggering OS 3.0 labeling off into loops of additional narratives. We often have judgments attached, showing themselves in OS 4.0 awareness—heightened attention and attraction to the positive feelings, rejection or dulled-out avoidance of others: judgment by mindlessness, in essence. These reactions are often imprinted and reinforced early in life, more indelibly in dysfunctional family ecosystems.

Getting to know one's own feeling states gets even more tricky when some of them are historically banned as off-limits to self-inquiry. "No one was allowed to be angry in our house" creates a distorted judgment, and we may even try to deny subsequent, valid grievances in order to avoid feeling that dreaded emotion. Witnessing unrelenting sadness in a chronically depressed parent can groove in a fear that today's brief, passing blues is just a baby step from a (OS 1.0) collapse into that deeper pain. But these experiences are exactly what to examine, carefully and with self-compassion.

Everything in mind, whether on the cushion or not, is "novel" at first, including emotions, and can initially generate a perceived increase in intensity because of that novelty. It's that split second in the cold pool before one gets used to the water. That initial burst can quickly induce deep survival fear, the dreaded "collapse to 1.0" that can add to or even overwhelm the feeling state. Even intense physical and emotional sensation is aided by not contributing to it and learning by serial experience that these states truly come and go. Only the observing awareness—our "home" to come back to—keeps hanging around, ready for the next wavicle bump in the field.

We'll work with a couple of practices specifically on emotions, including use of a helpful meteorological metaphor I employ in teaching youngsters, as well as a series of "subtle energy" areas of the body, known historically in Eastern medicine as "chakras," to tune into both the physical and the associated emotional aspects of the moment. My surgeon friends from medical school would tell you they've never excised a third chakra or lanced an inflamed sixth one, as they chortle behind their masks. On the other hand, my veteran meditator friends generally roll their eyes at the surgeon types who refuse to appreciate a level of felt experience that can't easily be measured (and doesn't require anesthesia or masks). Vive la différence. For me, I'm a "chakra agnostic," but leaning in humility toward a sense of something of real value there.

Over to Dirk with the Weather

A metaphor that I concocted initially in teaching elementary school kids actually is pretty effective for anybody, regardless of age. Emotionality is a changing aspect of the field much like the day's weather. While they can impact the whole body, historically we tend to associate emotions with, or even "locate" them in the torso—the anxious gut, the passionate heart. Practice with the kids involves imagining a window on one's own chest, looking in on the weather there, like one would check for angry thunderclouds, joyous sun, rainy sadness, or a chilly, anxious day. The practice slyly helps with the dual aspects of both being immersed in a state of emotion yet also observing it, looking through that window.

With mastery of emotion as an object of observation, we can include it as part of the daily routine like the short form of the body scan or as the main event in the work. It can also be the "audible" that gets called when that emotion is yanking attention away from whatever else is the intended target and needs "dropping into."

Emotions Practice No. 1: Look Through a Window, What Do You See?

The emotional "weather" of the moment, whatever that feeling state is, that's the object of observation here. You can practice this way:

- Settle and prep with HWG... (the intention is to open to my emotional "weather").

- Warm up with breath work, some reps of watching/losing/regaining attention, and a brief body scan; "breathe into them," if you like that tactic.

- With that feeling stable-ish, then pivot to observation of your emotional tone. You can simply attend to, "how am I feeling right now?" You can also work the more imaginal route, visualizing a window into your heart and looking inward. Notice how it feels physically.

- It is natural to label the state you find (calm, angry, joyful, anxious, etc.)—that's ok. But resist running narratives about where from, why now, or other trails.

- Stick with this focus for short periods—a few minutes at a time, then relax back to the breath for a little while; then pivot back to watching the weather. Working slowly and carefully in "holding the emotion" in awareness is more important some heroic white-knuckling of an intense state.

- Be ready for attention to be gained and lost easily in this practice, especially at first. Whatever you got that day, do your best to attend to it. You can always move back "home" to the breath—that's fruitful practice, too.

- Close the practice in your familiar way: a move back briefly to the breath; then a letting go of any direction of awareness, just letting your mind be and resting back in the "watcher." There, we, are.

Emotions Practice No. 2: Today's Theme Ingredient Is...

Next, here's a twist we'll become more familiar with. Rather than waiting for and attending emotions to emerge, we can use memory and imagination to generate feeling states for examination. After whatever "warm-up" preliminary work you find helpful to get the ol' attentional motor running, you can then introduce a particular emotion of your choice for observation—like a "theme ingredient" on a TV cooking show. Which emotions to work with? Well, any and all. Grievance/anger, sadness, uncertainty/anxiety, directed fear, irritability are the main baddies. But don't just focus on those; engage the positive ones, too: peak joy, "satisfaction" or contentment, love, infatuation, excitement. And don't leave out working on situations or prompts that leave you mixed, or ambivalent, or unsure.

This works best by first culling memory for a ripe experience that is associated with a particular feeling state. Remember a hug from grandma, or your beloved dog being euthanized, or your first make-out session, or being fired for something you were wrongfully blamed for, or that breakup text from the person you thought truly cared. Or that make-out thing again. All of these, again, represent experiences born of interaction—that's a 2.0 thing we're working on, getting to know our own patterns in.

Another generator of emotion could be artistic or cultural. A photograph, movie, or a piece of music or art that reliably pushes an emotional button can be used. Any of these "triggers" or prompts can be introduced just before you start.

With that introduction, try practicing in this way:

- Familiarize yourself with the prompting content (memory, photo, etc.) that generates a particular emotional tone.

- HWG... (my intention is to open to some planned emotional "weather") and warm up with some basic breath, "pitch/catch," and body scan work.

- Then bring in the "theme." Attend to the emotion, "look in the window," or "breathe into" the one that you've chosen. Call it to mind and let it do its

● thing to you, asking, "how does this make me feel, right now?"

● The job here is bare observation of that emotion—how it feels in the body, what thought narratives it generates, and the extent it alters the sense of clarity of the field and the watching. What's the weather doing?

● As before, when aware of getting caught in chatter, catch and release. Move back to the anchor of the breath for a little bit, and then back out to the body, then back to the emotional "theme." Watch how the state ebbs and flows.

● As with the other emotions practice, it's best to work with the "theme" for short periods—a few minutes at a time at most, then relax back to the breath, then pivot back to watching that particular weather front you've chosen.

● Close the practice in your familiar way: to the breath; then a letting go of any direction of awareness, resting back in the "watcher." There, we, are.

This practice is a first real immersion into witnessing a fuller experience of those pattern sets we will expand upon: physical, emotional, and thought, immersed in the field. While attention to physical states is a relatively clean matter of directing awareness to a part, emotions are different: cultivated by events, and thus pretty much always attached to some conceptual content to be observed. Emotions practices work to isolate out the body/heart aspect for fuller focus.

Yet for some, especially attending to emotions may feel too overwhelming or ominous to approach, especially in working with traumatic events, the risk of "collapse to 1.0," a deep goo of depression and/or agitation can feel threatening and not worth the effort. Here's where working with a teacher or psychotherapist with an understanding of these practices can help in supporting and guiding you, even advising you away from working with certain states or content in this way. There are plenty of other ways meditation training can help you if this particular practice is more painful than it is enlightening.

Chakras Can (Lemme Love 'Em...)

Next up is sketching out a basic exercise using those presumed, "subtle body" energy centers, known as chakras, as a fruitful construct for weaving body and emotion together in one practice. You may or may not have some familiarity via yoga or acupuncture with this perceived energy, referred to variously as ch'i, qi, or prana. It's above my pay grade to provide an exacting description of the highly complex literature on this subject. A few billion individuals over the millennia who have tended to their awareness in this manner provide some validation for making our own use of it here, even as the supposed energy flow doesn't move a needle or show up distinctly on a PET scan.

This energy doesn't wreak havoc in Heisenbergian improbability, bouncing off the spleen and lodging in the left eustachian tube. It follows (yet another) map—a "central channel" traveling along the spinal canal from the keister to out the top of head. Along that central path are seven nodes—the "chakras" themselves—each of which is associated with both a physical area of the body and an identified, linked emotional tone commonly felt there. Not that surprisingly, the channel includes a "mind's eye" node correlative with the pre-frontal cortex, our speculative center of 4.0 awareness, before exiting out the "crown" chakra atop the head.

The chakra system seems like a page out of an electrician's manual—describing circles of energy flow, running up and down the channel as well as cylindrically around the body and with potential "blockades" interrupting energy flow at those seven nodes if unattended to. My sensitivity to subtle changes in energy in my own carcass is not a fine-tuned instrument and probably never will be, but it has sharpened over time. With practice, it's an efficient way of getting your local self up and running, akin to flipping each light on and taking a brief (or longer) look around down the hallway of home.

A compassionate, cautionary note is order, guarding against what might be comically called "chakra shaming." Some folks, especially those deeply suspicious of Western medicine or prone to New-Agey simplifying, can overreach on the impact of this chakra thing, blaming physiologic suffering on a lack of proper attendance to energy "blocks." For example, I've worked with some patients who, demoralized by the lack of resolution of a difficult, chronic GI illness like Crohn's Disease or Irritable Bowel Syndrome, latch onto the distorted notion that they must carry blame for a lack of flow in their third or "gut" chakra. I myself have received supposedly some well-intended but ultimately accusatory, "your sixth (throat) chakra problems caused your cancer" speculations from some acquaintances. Thanks, I guess. Again, uncertainty must prevail.

I'll instead summarize with nicknames, locations and associated emotional states and sufferings thereof, for you to internalize them easily and use them fruitfully. Once familiar, we can use this variation to bringing attention to the physical and emotional in tandem assessing for blocks and tune-outs too.

- First Chakra/"*Root*": located in the region of your pelvic floor/base of spine/anal sphincter, this node is associated with "rootedness"—safety, security, and nourishment—or the lack thereof. It's deeply reflected in 1.0: a sense physically of lack of tension and emotionally of safety when things are ok, and of tension and deep insecurity emotionally in the "1.0 collapse" state.

- Second Chakra/*"Need/Pleasure"*: this chakra is located slightly north, generally felt in one's genitals. The physical association here is with carnal sensation, and the emotional tone tending toward need fulfillment. It's sometimes described as the "center of creativity," perhaps to link it with pro-creation, but confuses the issue with other aspects of creative experience. To me, creativity is more of a chakra orchestra—the heart's passion, the voice's expression, the brain's conceptual generation, etc. Trouble here is reflected in a felt sense of primal feeling, craving, and/or depressive emptiness.

- Third Chakra/*"Gut"*: this well-identified node is physically associated with your "gut"—the mid-abdomen. In a positive emotional sense, this chakra is identified with assuredness, self-confidence. Difficulties thereof follow as the opposites of those: uncertainty, anxiety, under-confidence, a felt sense of powerlessness.

- Fourth Chakra/*"Heart"*: this chakra is perhaps the most easily located of all, in the upper chest and encompassing the breath and heartbeat. The Sanskrit term for the node, "*anahata*," is usually translated as "unstruck" or "unhurt," pointing aspirationally to a pure center or core of the self underneath suffering and reactivity. The emotional tones associated here are the experience of openness, compassion, and empathy. In positive activity, "passion" is identified with the heart chakra. Suffering experiences of anger, grievance, sadness, and even hatred are associated with energetic difficulties.

- Fifth Chakra/ *"Voice"*: Moving northward from the intuitive "gut" through the passionate "heart," this node, located at the throat, emphasizes expression. It's associated emotionally, in my mind, with the self's sincere expression of truth. A sense of mattering is centered here, communicating new wavicles of value. The emotional difficulties associated with devaluing, having one's experience limited or muffled, can manifest in this area.

- Sixth Chakra/ *"Head"*: This chakra is located in the "third eye" spot, between and behind the eyes. It's associated, of course, with the intellect, wisdom, and (meta-)awareness. Struggles or blockades in the chakra range from the "blizzard brain" of mental chatter to a sense of slowing or even drying up of mental energy.

- Seventh Chakra/ *"Crown/Up and Out"*: This uppermost node is located at the very crown of the head, where the infant fontanelle once existed in baby days. It represents an exit point for the free flow of subtle energy through the central channel and out, into the field outside the locally perceived self. Its associations are often spiritual and metaphysical ones, the energetic intersection of Vibe and constructed, separate self. Common drawings depict energy spewing out the top of the head like a fountain and cascading around the physical self and back in below, forming a doughnut-shaped "torus" field enveloping the physical self. While this flow-shape of energy may or may not have some palpable relevance in your practice, it can be a useful visualization—pulling the energy of attention inward with the in-breath through the root chakra, up and out through the crown chakra.

That's a lot of mapping and identifying to do. Let's try to simplify:

- Root: your butt; security, insecurity
- Sex: your privates; needs and pleasures, met or unmet
- Gut: your abdomen; confidence, anxiety, uncertainty, sadness
- Heart: your chest; passion, compassion, heartache, grievance
- Voice: voice box; expressing, mattering, being understood
- Head: behind your eyes; thinking, awareness, chatter, empty head
- Crown and Out: "central path" out the top of your head; connection, or lack thereof

In developing a feeling for this exercise, it may be worth a little pre-sitting review with this summary in front of you, locating each area, cheating a peek at the body areas and associated emotional tones. Over time, each combo will become familiar. As you may surmise, this "chakra trail" nicely integrates aspects of the physical map and the OS framework in one practice.

It's more or less inevitable that some heavy storytelling may occur in this practice—emotions and their physical correlates are often deeply reactive targets. As you become aware of getting caught in those, "catch and release," move back to the anchor of the breath for a little bit, and then back out to the to the node as tolerated. Watch the ebbs and flows.

As with the other emotions practice, it's best to work with each node for short periods—a few minutes at a time at most, then relax back to the breath, then try again pivoting back to watching it again, or moving along.

With that introduction, try practicing in this way:

- Settle into a comfortable position; prep: Here, We, and...Go (the intention is to open to a sequential observation of the chakras and their associated physical and emotional attributes). Warm up as per your routine—breath, reps, body, out to field.

- When you're ready, direct your attention to the base of your spine and the first chakra. Observe the physical experience of your "root," witnessing any heaviness, tightness, discomfort, or perhaps attention pulling away. (As before, inhale to "gather awareness," then "breathe into" the area, if that tactic helps).

- As you feel the space physically, also note your sense of basic safety and security—its presence or absence, and whether it pulls you off into distraction. If so, resettle back into HWG, a recentering breath or two, and back to the chakra—physical sensation, linked emotional association. Stick with it for a few minutes.

- Next, move your attention to the second chakra. Observe the physical experience of your genital area, witnessing, for instance, a sense of sexual or other craving, or perhaps any dullness of that. Like with the prior exercises, "breathing into" the area may be a useful, if awfully weird sounding, tactic.

- As you observe, also note your sense of sensory satisfaction and fulfillment versus need or deprivation—basic presence or absence. As always, try to have an eye out on the "meta" quality—what lures you off into distraction. If/when that occurs, reset and back to the chakra—physical sensation, linked emotional association. Stick with it for a few minutes.

- Moving one more step up the chain, place your attention on your upper abdomen—your "gut." Witness it physically—noises, grumbles, discomfort, fullness, reflexive tightness, whatever you find. Also attend to the emotional tone: what is your "gut" telling you right now?

- This is a region that often signals uncertainty and anxiety versus a self-confident centeredness with the current moment. Self-judgment often collides with any other observation of the emotional self and registers here as fear that the moment can't or won't be tolerated. Watch for that possible patterning—physical, emotional, judgmental—as common in this area. Take it in short stretches as tolerated, returning to basic breath work, then back into the gut.

- When you're ready, move to the fourth or "heart" chakra. This is most familiar from basic practices in meditation on the breath and the heartbeat, easy to "breath into" and out of. As you hold it in attention, check the emotional "weather" there—of passion, power, connection. It also may be an intense but uncomfortable feeling state—anger or the "heartache" of sadness. You may note an absence—a muffled or blunted sense of emotion. Note whatever is there, tied to the physical state of the area.

- Next, move up to your neck—the voice or throat node. If it helps, imagine the exhaled breath moving up and thru the throat. Note relaxation or tension in the voice box and neck muscles. As you observe that physical sensation, attend to the familiar emotional associations here—expression, making oneself understood, communicating out into the wavicle field in a positive sense. Be aware of possible absence—a perception of being unheard, silenced, not valued and accepted. Don't imagine, just note what you find.

- Upward with a few breaths, focus your attention on a spot inside your cranium, just up from and behind your eyes. Place attention there and scan around inside the room a little. Note the physical attributes of your skull and its contents. Feel full inside? Spacious? Numb? Is there a headache? Is there a blizzard of thoughts? Leave a deeper examination of those for another sitting—just note them now. Instead, tend to the familiar emotional associations of this chakra—observe a sense or quality of your awareness itself, and of body/heart/mind coherence or lack thereof, or anything in between. Take your time in sitting to become familiar with the physical and emotional felt sense from this "vantage point," as it will be fruitful in our subsequent work in sitting in "4.0."

● Move onward to the last node, the crown chakra. A favored approach here is to focus on a sense of release—visualize of energy and attention gathered in each in-breath and exhaled out of the crown of the head to connect to the broader field of awareness around. The associated emotional felt state is a sense of belonging, of connection. Those with strong faith practices may find this a useful variation on a sense of relationship to a higher power, for other individuals, to cherished loved ones. If the practice feels forced, that's ok—observe experience, do not manufacture it.

● Consider integrating an additional tactic: cycling breath in creating that enveloping sense of a field around the physical self. You may visualize energy and attention pulled in via the central channel with the in-breath, pausing for a snapshot of emotional tone, and exhaling out and into the field with the out-breath—in a sense bringing your awareness to the whole of you, physically and emotionally, in one practice. It's all there to note without need for judgment or storytelling. As with the other exercises, be patient, work for a little while, and then take breaks back to basic breath work.

● Close the practice in your familiar way: a move back briefly to the breath, "coming up for air," then a letting go of any direction of awareness, just letting your mind be and resting back in whatever arises. And, voila: There, we, are.

The script above is long and kind of complicated, detailed in order to provide a full walk-through. You may choose to just work with a single chakra at a sitting; consider that as an incremental way of learning ad internalizing the physical and associated emotional aspects. Or work your way through all of them. Don't be surprised if one or more particular nodes are "hot" (with an intense or full sense of reaction) or "cold" (routinely dull, numb, or muted in experience). That could mean something; it generates invites the courageous to go back there, at your own pace and choice, for a closer look.

Summary: Emotions in Motion

We've covered a span of approaches to getting in better touch with the ever-changing states of emotion of a life lived moment to moment. After reiterating a warm-up routine, we worked on attending to whatever emotion is identifiable in the current moment, using "weather" as a useful metaphor. We varied the practice by employing an imaginal tactic, working to voluntarily "generate" an emotional state to sit with via memory or media in order to access and observe what happens, including how other reactions can follow. We finished with a dive into a kind of combined practice of body and heart, of physical and emotional phenomena, using the historically significant "map" of subtle energy work involving chakras. The purpose in this admittedly more involved, complicated exercise is to animate a more thorough, linked "survey" of both body and emotion.

I suggest you incorporate them into a regular sequence of:

- *an introductory, anchoring warm-up ("HWG," breath, body check-in)*

- *pivoting to the "Go" intention of your choosing—"what's on today" attending to the emotional weather of the moment, or a "serve it up" generating of an emotional state, or practicing with one or all of the chakras (nodes with both physical and emotional attributes to observe for)*

- *make good use of that "breathing into" tactic*

- *anticipating (and watch your self-judgment about) the inevitable losses of attention and keeping a "meta" eye on what might be driving those disruptions*

- *closing with a letting go of effort, resting back in the watcher (and with an eye out for what happens to attention), and then a closing routine ("TWA")*

I dropped a hint earlier about thoughts being their own special thing. We love our thoughts. We can be entranced by them. Let's work next on attending to them.

CHAPTER 10

"I Think" Becomes, "There's That Thought"

The next set of practices in taming the wild wavicles of experience has the humble aim of loosening that death grip on the pervasive outlook of "I am what I think." We grow quite attached to and identify with "our" thoughts deeply, even as "they" truly come and go like sensations, emotions, clouds, and lapel widths.

We've established that a thought, like a kick in the shin or a reaction to a friend's smile, is but another species of wavicle event frolicking in the field of momentary experience. Like other events, we tend to reflexively react to the thought and then ritually judge that reaction. That thought/reaction/judgment can get recycled without examination. A couple hundred thousand replays of that process later, the whole blur eventually becomes its own perceived "truth" by and about the individual. A fixed, hard-to-shift temperament and outlook can result.

Ironically, the most distorted views of self can be the most difficult, even threatening, to change. It would represent a big alteration to the current, familiar landscape of mind. "I'm not the idiot I always default to labeling myself when I make even a tiny mistake? Who am I, then?" "My proud sense that I'm 'just speaking the truth' to others is actually me being controlling and pushy? Why, that can't be so…

can it?" These novel revelations—new emanations of the 3.0 thinky mind—are hard to hold, challenging to allow in, but worth a deep look to reduce their influence.

I'd opine that fully divorcing oneself from any identification with the thought content popping up in one's field is but pretty much impossible on an ongoing basis. But, aiming a little lower, it is altogether doable to start relaxing the white-knuckled grasp on a pervasive, "that thought is me."

Thought Stopping (That's a Thought Worth Stopping)

Cognitive/behavioral training often focuses on thoughts as enemy combatants, directing people to try to "stop" them, like some wavicle citizen's arrest, when a rogue thought inevitably invades the field. Thoughts can subside for some moments or brief stretches of time, but getting thoughts to stop, short of anesthesia or a shuffle off the mortal coil? Nope.

This comically unrealistic ideal sets the individual up for not just the struggle of pesky thoughts inevitably defeating the idealized "stopping," but also for some unnecessary, additional self-criticism (ironically, more thoughts to feel bad about!) Further, when we bluntly try to "stop the thought," we leave that paper trail of our fuller, more complex patterns of reaction undiscovered, and thus more prone to persistence. So, let's dispense with silly thoughts about stopping thoughts.

Let's approach it first with some humble acceptance regarding our workings of mind: thoughts happen. They are a condition of consciousness, coming and going in awake moments and while asleep, too. There are certainly moments, both in and out of meditative practice, of a clarity of the field, with stretches of time with little-to-no perceived thoughts in the way. For some, this is blissful, for others, a little creepy and fearsome, at least at first. And then, inevitably, mind pops another idea, or memory, or speculation, like whack-a-mole. Short of unplugging the damn machine, the moles keep popping up.

Instead, meditation actually involves the intentional observation of thoughts, or moles, or any other wavicle, subsiding or not, in and as part of the field. That's it. We can aim to manage our attention to thoughts as they arise and disperse spontaneously, and we can attend to the reaction generated. We try not to let a spontaneous thought "spin" up quick-trigger, familiar cascades of physical and emotional reactivity, and knee-jerk judgmental narratives. My favored punchline to patients struggling with this aspect of meditation is, "give the thought a seat at the table, but you keep running the meeting."

I Think...I'll Just Rent

One other outlook-shifting approach involves ownership. Physical sensations come and go, as do emotional feeling states, states of awareness, and, of course, thoughts. Nevertheless, the recurrent, even ritual nature of thinking, cycling like a Maytag stuck on "spin cycle," can lead us to a personal identifying with the thoughts occurring in the field, and a misperception that we possess them, take ownership of them.

Thoughts also come and go. Like all the other stuff, they are impermanent. The only real persistent, sustained player in the field of mind is the observer. More accurately from a quantum viewpoint, it's the *observing*—the interaction.

Eschewing thought "ownership," we can opt instead for a kind of short-term rental. None of the upcoming practices with thoughts run the fool's errand of trying to stop them. Instead, we'll work with them, transcend and tolerate them when we must, and examine them when we can or wish to.

First, we'll work with a familiar "catch and release" kind of practice. Thoughts can pop up as a distraction or even defense during any meditation, so having a way of managing the moles is a useful tool. One variation will involve basic noting and return, the other a slight bit more tuned into the "meta" thing before returning to the prior intention of the session.

Then we'll treat thoughts to actual, explicit attention and observation, using our maps and looking for those pattern sets. Thoughts often emanate from the subconscious as cryptic clues to feeling states or as defensive distractions. They can represent reactions to other events and, maybe especially, judgments on other thoughts or feelings.

So lastly, we'll work two slightly more complicated practices: closely examining thoughts and what piece they may be in the puzzle of the moment, and turning to the "meta" quality of the observing itself.

Thoughts Practice No. 1: Catch and Release

The basic tactic of this practice can be used with any of the other practices of breath, body, or emotion we've already covered; for simplicity's sake, let's use basic breath meditation. That's the object of observation here, with the intention to return to that basic practice when any thought distraction arises.

You can practice this way:

- Settle and warm up with HWG (my intention is to watch my breathing and thoughts that intrude). Consider ten to twenty minutes for this practice, aside from any warming up period (set a timer if that helps).

- Settle as usual into a pattern of observation by letting the breath move to its natural state, whatever that is. You may use a bare observation or the three-point practice (in, out, "landscape out" to a check of body sensation).

- Inevitably, you will notice a thought or thoughts, whether coexisting with your attentional focus, or even pulling at your attention to examine and "work on." As you become aware of that, turn attention briefly but directly to attend to the thought and acknowledge it. Do that simply, without fuss, perhaps with a brief, internal memo to self: "there's a thought."

- Then release your attention from its brief, deliberate shift to the thought "wavicle" and return to the plan—watching the breath. If a voluntary reset of "HWG" helps in the return to your intended practice, go ahead.

- One additional tactic can be helpful: just after noting the thought, pull attention back to full "landscape mode"—briefly witnessing the thought as a part of subset of a larger field of "here and now." Then, back to the breath.

- Proceed with attention inevitably impacted by thought phenomena. Catch, note, and release the thought, striving to avoid elaborating on it; briefly pull back and see it as one-bit player in the field; and return to breath.

- At the end of your period of practice (i.e. when the timer sounds) close the practice in your way: a letting go of any direction of awareness for a bit, just letting your mind be; rest back in the "watcher." There, we, are.

For those with a cooking background, think of this practice as a "mother sauce." Let's tweak it into remoulade.

Thoughts Practice No. 2: Drop and Roll with It

You may have observed that the tactic laid out above would be a good tool to use with any phenomena of experience that are dominating or photobombing your session's practice intention—not just with thoughts.

You'd be right. You can directly "turn attention into" a distracting body sensation or emotional input as a way of firmly, deliberately noting that current aspect of the field in mind, and then directing attention back to your initial intention. Thoughts just tend to be a really sticky, common distractor, so I'm emphasizing it here. But feel free to use it here, and there and everywhere.

Thoughts can sometimes be so sticky that a simple "catch and release" tactic is not enough to shed them. Furthermore, they could actually be intruding with some useful purpose.

So, this variation on the first exercise adds a familiar tactic: *"dropping into"* the concurrent somatic and emotional tone that may be riding along with the distracting thought or thought patterns. If the thought(s) is/are persistently intrusive, there may be some impact on the other OSs, enough to warrant a check. It's a good excuse for practicing opening out to a broader "aperture," using the opportunity to witness a fuller "pattern set" of thought/emotion/sensation, all of the OSs playing, that a blizzard of thoughts often serve to defend.

One other good reason for dropping into the rest of the local experience and rolling in it: "meta" practice. We're getting some reps in practicing our awareness in various ways, which inevitably walks us back to becoming more familiar with the driver's seat of the watcher.

Observation here remains on the breath with the intention to return to that basic practice when any thought distraction arises—but with some more directed tactics to work with when those thoughts inevitably barge in.

You can practice this way:

- Settle and warm up with HWG (my intention is to watch my breathing and "drop into" thoughts as they intrude). Let the breath move to its natural state and proceed with breath observation.

- When the experience of an intrusive thought eventually presents itself, turn directly in attention to that thought or set of recurrent ideas. Take a breath, stabilizing your attention on this new, specific target. "Breathe into it" as a kind of interaction with this aspect of your current mindscape.

- Then, make the drop—open to how it feels physically, then emotionally. It can help to imagine "contracting" attention around the thought with your in-breath, then "breathing it out" into your body and observe for the bodily experience; gathering it up in attention with the next in-breath, and then "breathing it into" the heart for a snapshot of the emotional impact.

- Watch what changes over a little bit of time of that dropping into the body and heart. When you open to the physical feeling or emotional tone, do the thoughts drop away? Do they crank up? Do you lose attention completely?

- Explore the whole pattern—body, heart, and thought—for a short period, a minute or two at most; then drop back to a reset and back to your initial intention of observing the breath. With any

> subsequent "thought intrusions," again "drop into" the set of thoughts and associated physical and emotional experience, gathering awareness in the in-breath, and releasing it to your observation in the out-breath.
>
> 💬 Close the practice like usual: a short period of letting go of any direction of awareness, just letting your mind be and resting back in the "watcher," the meta-mind. There, we, are.

Be ready for and humble about the inherent challenge of this practice, especially at first. You are working on some more complex shifts—from breath, to thoughts, to their associated physical and emotional aspects, and the inevitable (4.0) attentional losses and restarts. Be patient and nonjudgmental as best you can.

Thoughts Practice No. 3: Theme Ingredient Redux (A Thought Wavicle, or a Whole Blizzard of Them)

Next in this series on working with thought phenomena in the field of mind, we'll use a tactic from the last chapter on emotional states, deliberately introducing a thought or pattern of thoughts as a target for observation, as opposed to waiting for one to emerge. It's useful to have that target selected at the outset before you begin. The target can be a solitary conceptual wavicle, from a simple or trivial one—hair, potatoes, Velcro, autumn—to a complex and/or provocative one, such as joy, death, sex, war, pain, gratitude. It may be a particular thought that's been bugging you all week, or a recent interpersonal interaction that perhaps reminds you of something older and familiar. It's all fair game.

The hitch is in what to intend to do, and not do, with that thought wavicle. This practice is not intended as "analysis," not about thinking about the thought(s)—though that will likely happen. Instead, it's intended as radical, bare observation of the target thought— introducing and holding the idea in mind, and then observing what happens in the field, locally (inside the skin) and beyond. Does it generate a comfortable physical feeling? Vague nausea? Some surprising anger? A shift to a separate, maybe "safer" subject in terms of distracting, alternative thoughts? Or maybe there's nothing—just dullness? We cast our mind's eye with some thought bait, and then closely watch for some drama to unfold through the OSs. We catch and release what gets generated and keep moving back to the watcher and the watching.

This exercise is admittedly difficult, as thoughts tend to beget more thinking, reacting, and judgment. In that regard, the "dropping into" aspect, opening to body and feeling, is a really helpful one in this practice. We're literally planting a thought seed in the field of mind, then watching what reactive elements might grow somatically and emotionally. Beyond those two realms, what happens in terms of further 3.0 narrative (i.e. additional thinking), and more subtly in the clarity and stability of the 4.0 attention, are also worthy of observation.

Through repetition, we gain some familiarity with those "pattern sets"—linked phenomena of body/heart/mind/awareness that get generated by particular thoughts, often in a predictable way. We become less surprised at their showing up and learn to moderate and even dissipate our reflexive reactions. This awareness generates better control and adaptation.

Which thoughts to work with? Well, like with emotions, any of them. Engage single and complex ones, positive and negative ones. Much of the time, my own daily practice includes "theme ingredient" time, opening to a "ripe" situation or dilemma. The "soundtrack" of associated body, heart, and attention effects unfolds with the presentation, ready to be dropped into. Attention is lost and gained; sometimes familiar patterning emerges for noting; sometimes some new awareness of an aspect of my patterning bubbles up. And sometimes it's just crickets. You get what you get.

With that introduction, try practicing this way:

- Settle and warm up with HWG (my intention is to introduce and work with a thought). Let the breath move to its natural state and proceed with some breath observation. Shake the rust off your awareness.

- With that feeling stable-ish, then bring in the "theme thought." "Declare" it, then back off to a bare observation of its effect—how it feels in the body, what emotional feelings may bubble up, what further narratives it generates, any way it alters the sense of clarity of the field and the watching. Feel free to utilize that "dropping /breathing into" tactic set to help ground the experience.

- It's normal to identify the qualities that emerge. It's inevitable that some "storytelling" (more thoughts) may occur and lead to getting lost and distracted. Use your skills—note, easy on the judgment, reset via a move back to the anchor of the breath and body for a little bit, and then back out to the "theme thought" as tolerated.

- Repeat and reintroduce the theme in your field, then watch how the state ebbs and flows. Work with the "theme thought" focus for short periods—a few minutes at a time at most, then relax back to the breath, then try again.

> 💬 Close the practice in your familiar way: a move back briefly to the breath; then a letting go of any direction of awareness, just letting your mind be and resting back in the "watcher." There, we, are.

Another cautionary note: as with the practice involving voluntary introduction of emotions, this practice may feel *too overwhelming with 1.0 suffering for some to approach or stick with.* That can happen if known traumatic material is voluntarily tackled; getting a feel for what to dive into becomes a matter of self-regulation, of pragmatic care, and usually of some consultation with a teacher. Again, there are plenty of other ways this training can help you if a particular practice such as this feels unhelpful or worse.

There is also the possibility that a perceived-as-unprovocative thought, introduced as a "theme" for observation, springs open a flood of intense other stuff including traumatic memories and feelings. In that case, it's absolutely ok to back off, settle back into the breath and body, or stop the exercise. The intentional ground of the practice is compassionate care for the self, not some tortured gauntlet.

It bears reiteration that such "collapse" (or close) events are real red flags to get some consultation with a meditation teacher and/ or psychotherapist.

The opposite trend to become more aware of is an "exit stage left" effect with certain thoughts. This can be of the jittery monkey-mind variety or just a dulling out that happens each time the thought is presented in mind. Both types of reactions may just be an aspect of the day and the meditator, but could also mean that there is something important, uncomfortable, or both about the theme.

Watching the quality of the observing in this way, that's developing "meta" in action. That process bears its own sequence to review.

Thoughts Practice No. 4: Heavy Meta

As we get into more complex exercises, the in-the-moment decision-making about dropping in, resting back, and other tactics becomes more apparent as an aspect of the work. This meta-awareness, this "little me on my shoulder," attending to the observing as it proceeds, is an ongoing, parallel process aspect of OS 4.0 that we're training all along. The directed "resting in the observer, observing" is something that you may have noticed I've been sneaking in, like kale in the family lasagna recipe, at the end of sessions to let the directed mind relax out to whatever's happening, but to observe what happens with that release. This last thought practice is a more specific way to work with that meta.

With that introduction, try practicing in this way:

- Settle in (HWG...the intention is to open to how a particular thought affects my observing experience). Practice a bit on the breath to warm up.

- With that feeling stable-ish, then bring in the "theme thought," as we've learned. Present in mind an idea, then backing off as before to a bare observation of its effect in the body, feelings, and further thought.

- Here's the shift: with some stability in observing that pattern set of introduced thought and its associations and reactions, place your attention on the watching itself. What is quality of that view? Does it get more scattered? Duller, like a dirty windshield? More intense? Or does the generator start to flicker? Observe how the object of attention alters the sense of clarity of the field and the watching.

- Work with the "meta" or "watching the watcher" focus for short periods—a few minutes at a time.

Then rest back in the familiar, such as breath or body practice. Then back out to the work, as tolerated.

● Close the practice in your familiar way: a move back briefly to the breath; then a letting go of any direction of awareness, just letting your mind be and resting back in a more relaxed observation of the field. There, we, are.

As a whole, this practice wades into a fuller experience of pattern sets: physical, emotional, and now thoughts, and the watching itself—all there to be attended to. Ultimately, this exercise works on the reality of our being immersed in the broadest view: moment after moment of an observer interacting with our whole field of observation, including the observing and observer.

Braving the Blizzard (Turn Off the Snow-Makers!)

We've covered a sequence of practices attending to the most likely distractors in the moment-to-moment field of consciousness— thoughts, and our thoughts about them. It's harder to examine the patterning that dances around these things, whether in the body and heart, or in additional thinking, when we clutch too tightly to each thought as a desperately held possession. Putting down the psychic label makers we reflexively use to label thoughts as, "Property of: Me" can become more routine. Besides the "rent it, don't own it" admonition, please question the widely held silliness that we can stop thoughts from arising.[45] It's what we do with them that matters most.

From those basic precepts, we rolled into a series of exercises that hopefully are becoming familiar in sequence and style:

---

45 Or ocean waves, or the weather, or more Kardashians. They keep coming. That's just science.

- A no-frills *"breathe and watch what happens"* practice emphasizing not grabbing onto thoughts and running new narratives, but instead briefly noting and the returning to the prior plan. "Catch and Release" was the nickname.

- A similar "breathe and watch" practice, but with the additional rule of holding thoughts that come up just a little longer for *"dropping into"* before release, to observe associated bodily and emotional phenomena that may be running with the thought—"conditioned" with it.

- We took those sequences and worked on going right at particular thoughts rather than waiting for them to arise. The *"theme ingredient"* practice is applicable to other phenomena of the field of mind. Bringing "material" in for observation, even in imagination, is a useful complement to psychotherapy, journaling, and other forms of developing self-understanding and, ultimately, self-acceptance.

- Lastly, we went *"meta,"* pulling observation back to include the quality of the observing itself as thoughts and their reactive extras come and go. Getting a regular feel for, and gratitude for, this precious faculty is worth building into each phase of our practice.

We've covered a lot of ground so far. Let's take a literal moment or two to take stock of where we're at. We'll dig into some examples of how the maps and exercises can be used in some special moments of experience, both scheduled and unforeseen. Then, we'll set up for the last leg of our journey home.

CHAPTER 11

It's a Bee-you-tee-ful Day for Meditation!

For something as subjective as observing one's own mind in action, the "recipes" for practice only take an individual so far. While every "sitting" is a unique series of moments, providing a more extensive play-by-play of one such sitting could help things. Look for some sense of the routine, the obstacles, the tactics, and the bumps of mind in action; they may be similar to yours at one point or another. I'll break in at a couple of points to comment where useful.

A Wednesday morning, 8:04 a.m.,[46] my smartphone vibrating and playing a quiet Handel sonata[47] to remind me that it's time to stop fiddling with the billing software and meditate.

Settling onto the cushion, I wiggle a little until it feels right. It's a tad chilly in the office, so I use a small throw blanket I have around to cover my lap. No need to caress my face with it, thumb in mouth, but just a casual toss across my legs. Hands are palm down on thighs; my gaze trained lazily on a stubborn old coffee stain on my office rug—now a part of "home" in my practice, a little comic reminder of accepting imperfection as I sit.

---

46   A fussy habit of mine: I intend to be on the cushion at eight o'clock sharp; my phone goes off at 8:04 to shame me that I'm late. Probably something to analyze there.

47   Ironically, the lovely Handel piece is one I've struggled to master in my own piano practice; some symbolism for me there, every morning.

A little preparatory decision-making, right here: I've been pre-occupied this a.m. about a voicemail from a managed care company, "requesting a clinical peer review" for a fragile patient who's needed lots of care in the last six months. Such reviews can have value but often devolve into unilateral restrictions of treatment from another professional despite scant information on the case. I've been here before, as have most shrinks.

But it's set me off a bit. Even before "sitting with it," I have going on an interior, gooey mix of affront, chattering thoughts, and a soupçon of some kind of shame/guilt feeling. All of that, kind of swirling between the seven o'clock voicemail check and 8:04, makes it a good thing to work with today, nudging off the calendar my intended "watch what happens" practice plans.

You can customize make this practice your own and make skillful decisions to switch things up as circumstances arise.

Phone timer is set for fifteen minutes (twenty is all I got today, with a session at eight thirty in the morning), and I begin.

Here...belly breath number one, and with it a comforting, familiar construct of the field pops in. With the in-breath, the physical, emotional, thought, and awareness aspects of my sense of self in the moment. With the exhale, (I imagine exhaling out into the space around me, actually) an acknowledgment of the field in which I am immersed. (Sometimes I start here by imagining I'm flipping on the switches to each OS, like lights going on down a hallway. Mixing it up...)

We...wheeze number two, and with this in-breath, a nod to others striving to reduce their and others' suffering and become more aware, right now or whenever. Energy (imagined, literal, who knows?) from that "club" gets traded out, with gratitude, on the out-breath. A brief note that "we" includes the insurance representative I'll be tussling with. We all have our jobs to do.

Go...a third breath, and with it, setting my intention: some basic breath meditation to settle into the familiar "watch/lose it/get it back" mini-drama that is the core experience of this work; a brief body/emotion/ thoughts "scan" to flip on the attentional lights and examine further for whatever is or is not "simmering"; then, at some intuitive point, maybe five minutes in or so, switch to the "theme"—that gooey hairball of reactivity emanating from the morning call. When the timer sounds, I'll regroup for my usual closing, which includes a short period of compassion practice, a brief period of dropping back to "meta," and ending the sitting with TWA.

After HWG, I allow my breathing to do its own thing—arc up, arc down, out to the whole self at the bottom of the breath. This "trey" sequence is as familiar to me as starting my car. A little tight and contracted, it seems, then another, then...

The voicemail pops in as a vivid memory. Just after a tortured mispronunciation of my last name, it was a sugary, "we would appreciate a clinical review on your patient within the next three business days." A thought loop of the irony of the "we" and "your patient" juxtaposed, kicks in. A burst of grievance is felt in the chest; thoughts run toward a speechwriting stretch about power vs. responsibility and how I'll craft an inevitable appeal letter to that debate, and...yeah. I've gotten off track.

A little shame kicks up for how quickly the train got derailed, and then a smile—boy, I can get charged up! Chill, dude! A quick, reflexive "meta" check—why did that happen then?—yields nothing earth shattering; the badly botched pronunciation of my last name before the syrupy request smacked of insincerity, perhaps. I resettle, wiggling my ass to indicate a reset into position.

A nod is here to some inevitabilities: of the wavicle blizzard and of self-judgment that can kick up with the loss of smooth observation. I'm reinforcing the benefit of dropping the judge's gavel and taking a meta moment—use the breakdown and see if there is something to be learned. As for the "compassion practice," that's another book, but I'll describe an example here in this vignette.

A single deep breath, then back to arc up, arc down, stretch out. The flux of the call and my reactions waxes and wanes over the next few minutes. I consider a pivot into "turning into" it, as it is sort of lurking there, waiting to highjack things. But it's on the agenda, so I decide to stay on course. But mostly, I settle into a stable watching—breath, and "that s**t," kind of lingering, and some chest tension.

A couple of minutes pass and I proceed to a brief "OS scan"—gathering each in-breath, then releasing as attention to my bodily 1.0 self for a few breaths. I notice tension in my upper back muscles and that "heat," subtly, in the chest.

Then to emotional me, 2.0...and things go a bit awry. "Breathing into" my heart a couple of times reactivates the grievance, which triggers a thought association to the call, making me feel "radioactive," then that domino falls into a whole new line of thoughts, centered on my having actually had intensive radiation treatment for my malignancy fairly recently, for which I carry some ongoing, residual physical suffering. Then another domino, interior snark that this work stress is more lethal for me than the damn cancer or its treatment.

I stop. A quick "meta" check: mostly aware of the continuing presence of the voicemail-goo and how dropping into the body and heart pushed whatever it is into an unexpectedly darker place. And then some smiling at my inner melodrama.

This is a meaty moment in meditation—when a tactic opens up a blizzard of new wavicles in the field. New thought trails emerge and reactive emotions to those, too, some intense enough to generate secondary fear of overwhelm ("collapse to 1.0"). Skillful practice directs you to take it slow, reset; try to approach it carefully and deliberately, and with no shame in retreating to the safety of a more basic breath and/or body awareness practice, or even "done for now."

HWG...a couple of cycles of breath to stabilize this rocky sitting. I reengage the body and heart (a bit of careful, "oh, that again" with the radioactivity rant in memory), and then move to observe the state of OS 3.0 mind chatter. Opening to observation of the blizzard, I catch a thought pattern of "how dare they?" cycling with "they've trapped me, I've screwed up." Watch those thoughts, don't bite. The cycle persists— "dare" and "trapped" sharing space. My neck starts to ache, as if the tumor's got the mike. I decide to "drop into" the body and heart feeling coexisting with that chatter, and...

...into the tunnel I go. Awareness gets a bit fuzzy, tuned out; energy drops and I feel a little sleepy. It's like pudding up there. This goes on for a little stretch, maybe a couple minutes. Then, the "aha" kicks in, a mysterious thing—I've been gone and now back.

Resettling and some inquiry. A quick "meta" flash at "why tune out, then?" This is a familiar personal pattern—that "tune out" a kind of blanket thrown over dreadful thoughts of mortality. Amazing how "annoying insurance call" whispers down the lane and becomes "killer goober in my neck." But that's mind for you (or at least me, in that moment; you'll find your own patterns and links). The dread thing is an old acquaintance, challenging to engage but manageable.

This sequence captures the surprising shifts, from intensity to tune out, and the trusty "watcher" meta role that one can come home to and regroup with. As for the flashes of mortality...having stared into it many, many times with resultant settling of both the uncertainty I carry and the gratitude to be in a remission state. I make this sound easier than it's been.

A big deep breath and resettling there for a little bit. I introduce the "theme" which had already been primed by the preliminaries. I attend— again, but this time intentionally—to the voicemail, proceeding deliberately and carefully. I "drop into" what I witness in body, feelings, and further thought. The memory trace of the call regenerates a sinking feeling in the gut and some angry thought "scramble" upstairs. I stay disciplined: open to the memory, gather my attention and "breath into" an awareness of any effects, meta to staying observant to any quick pull offs into a new narrative rant or side issue.

The intensity of the whole thing softens with patient attending—it ain't the end of the world. The emotional two-step warbles: some anger, some guilt. The earlier, darker dive into survival fear seems to have resolved for now.

Some side narratives pop for me to catch and release. The prospect of the lawyerly preparing for clinical inquisition reveals a mix of anxiety, mostly felt in the gut, and a chest tight and hot with grievance at the extra work imposed and the chutzpah of the insurance monolith threatening to deny reimbursement, knowing little of my effort and worry. The grievance part is Velcro, easy to attach to the felt unfairness. I linger there a minute, breathing into the feeling state and occasionally needing to stop from storytelling enactments of the phone review to come. Best to change it up, pull back, rest, and observe from the watcher and then perhaps dive in again.

That other part needs observation—that failure feeling in the gut. Meta-me noted that change in my awareness itself, from chatter to tune out. It'd be a good thing to go there and see what happens.

Using the basic tools: settle and stabilize; look for meaning in the breaks in attention; drop into the body and heart to find out more; be careful, deliberate, curious, and try to resist the jury stuff; know you can come home to the observing you at rest whenever you need.

Resettle, a couple of breaths watched, then the other theme to open to: "trapped/screwed up." That theme gets quickly photobombed by a reprise of "those unfair a**holes!," experienced mostly in thought but with heart charging up again. Interesting. I stop, resettle, repeat. This, "guilty? no, be mad!" happens three or four more times, leading to a comic side-

conversation of "I'm in a 'lather'—rinse—repeat," which amuses me—my inner comedian a familiar distractor. Stop, again.

Back to a literal recitation of HWG to myself, and just settle with my breath for a bit, then... "trapped." The tune-out feeling kind of lurks, but I just hold "trapped" and observe. The heart and body go from tense and hot to...that other familiar pattern for me: trapped by illness, damaged, not whole. Some familiar associations flow...these daily tensions waste my time and that time is more precious than ever; some tension over trusting in the validity of my two years in remission; some residual distortion over tumor-as-cosmic-punishment; and some smiling eye-rolling over my unfinished business in handling this stuff.

The heart aches, but some understanding softens that, right there in real time. The grievance is of course still there, but that softens too; it feels less intense, less necessary to hold to. I pull back for a moment to "home," then "retest" each of these themes—"messed with" and "I'm trapped"—with some familiar returns of those patterns and reactions, but less intensely felt.

In the middle of one further "dive in," the timer goes off. The time passed feels in some ways like a blink of the proverbial eye, in another like an hour. But there's also a feeling of some fatigue—not a terribly relaxing, but fruitful piece of work on the cushion. I pull back to the breath and wrap up...

There...just let any direction of attention go and let it be, moving back to "meta" and sitting, observing the whole field. Moving back includes a check of the quality of the observing. How are things right now? Today, it doesn't jump me back into chatter, which sometimes can happen. I feel tired, but clear.

We... I proceed to a brief compassion exercise with the clock running away. I visualize my awareness as a manifestation of deep belonging, my membership in the Grand Society of Wavicles. This belonging noted, I take in a big, deep breath, and visualize the interactions I will have today, clinical and personal, and the suffering and difficulty, including my own, that come with that. With a slow out-breath, I visualize releasing an intention to be of help. I may repeat this for conviction.

Are...aware that I'm shifting from a more intense, inner-directed state of being to reentering the day-to-day. My right foot is asleep; I take a moment to let the blood flow return, and then get up and out into the day.

Granted, not every meditation session will have some of the twists and turns of the vignette above. But hopefully it provides some sense of the wide variety of what goes on in the field of mind. Next, we'll dig into handy tactics designed to manage some special moments of experience, both scheduled and unforeseen. After that, with a suite of meditation practices under our belts, we'll address some ideas on spreading the goodness of this practice.

CHAPTER 12

The Mind Hacker's Toolkit, for Those Special Moments

We've now covered the basics of starting a meditation practice: breath work, the gaining and losing and regaining of attention, then a survey of the physical, emotional, and thought aspects of mind. We'll ultimately proceed to exercises in attending to the full field of awareness, including the watching itself—out to the whole enchilada. But first, let's pause to take a few aspects of what we've already covered and apply them to some particular life moments where meditation could come in really handy.

The benefits of this work can come in fits and starts without any easy predictability of, say, the timing of a sense of improved clarity or the opening to a new interior understanding. Yes, it may sound a little like ol' Linus waiting in that damn patch for a grand squash. Yet there are a few tips worth reemphasizing to navigate the journey: some meditation "hacks," as the kids call 'em these days. These are tactics to have at the ready in figuring out patterning as it presents itself, to limit getting stuck in stretches of recurrent blizzards or tune-outs, and ultimately to reduce the risk of altogether bailing out on meditating out of sheer frustration.

After reiterating those go-to tools, we'll focus in on some special, challenging moments that having a brief meditative "recipe" at the ready can be very helpful for. As I elaborated on way back in Chapter 4, setting up optimal conditions for meditation is a good idea. But the settings and circumstances of a moment that could use some mindful attention are not always so optimal, or even close. They can be acute, maybe scary shifts in the momentary scene: abrupt anxiety, anger, or cravings for food or mind-bending "additives." We all have faced unexpected visitations of bad news or an unanticipated necessity to spring into action, performance, or caretaking. Interludes of resistance, boredom, or loss of motivation are less splashy events, but nevertheless can be intrusive and worth identifying, attending to, and moving off of. Other times, it's an unexpected gap in business or busy-ness that allows for an impromptu, brief "session," inviting us to take stock of the current mindscape. I'll provide some brief "band-aid" meditation exercises that most folks I work with find helpful.

Another category is more "vitamin" than "band-aid": intentional, scheduled routines prior to and/or after a workday, performance, or meeting, professional or personal. Preparatory tune in practices can generate a "fresh view" in engaging the next thing on the schedule. A sitting afterwards can give the moment its proper due in contemplation.

Don't Shoot the Trouble

It's understandable to long for the bliss and peace of a sustained settling of the experience of mind. If only that is how it usually unfolds. Heh.

Instead, the practice of meditation involves stretches of mindful and mindless experience, and some transitional states of entry/exit goo in between. With the shared aspiration of teacher (*moi*) and pupil (*vous*) to get you comfortable with the basics of meditating, it might seem appropriate to call this next lesson "troubleshooting." But I'd argue to spin it a different way.

In reality, we get lost in this practice so commonly that getting lost is not a bug, but actually a feature of meditation. We're witnessing the mind, and the mind gets lost. Mindlessness is not to be wished away, judged, or even longed for full protection from. (And, how boring it would ultimately be if we simply dropped into an absolute, ever-sustained clarity, with no struggle occurring ever again?)

So, an attitude readjustment about the uncertain experience of meditating is in order. Or disorder. Disorder in the observation of the mind is actually the steady state. What the sages call "presence," or sustained periods of alert-but-chill awareness, is a reasonable aspiration, but a somewhat unreasonable expectation, let alone an entitlement.

That's especially true in the way that most of us practice in the West—that is, with brief, prescribed periods of daily or routine sittings, and then busy lives to spring off the cushion into, lives of action and interaction. Outside of committing to longer stretches of meditative retreat in optimal conditions or even to meditation as a full-time lifestyle or career, a sustained, mindful state is just unrealistic. The metaphor of "I'll get up on these new skis, once down the bunny hill for practice, then off to the black diamond runs for me" is less apt than, well, surfing, or maybe even log rolling. You're gonna get wet.

Twenty years in, I love the bliss of my own intermittent moments of deeper meditative clarity. But, mostly, I expect to get wet, really wet. And with a ritual splash into mindlessness being an inevitability, it only makes sense to work on how to get back on the board, or log, or whatever. And we shall not give short shrift to what can be gleaned from the repeated dunking. It's all observable, all worthy of some more...shrift.[48]

---

[48] "Shrift" is actually an archaic term for "confession," an observation of lack of perfection. Yup.

That being said, let's go over those specific tactics in managing the inevitable ins and outs of clearer awareness.

Press Command-M, Then...

When attention becomes lost, there is a moment of "gone" and then, eventually, one of, "back again." In that return, there's an opportunity; but for many of us, that's the cue for some reactive "piling on" of self-judgment and critique. This usually adds little of benefit to the practitioner. Indeed, it's just another distractor.

Instead, we can follow the sweet recognition of mindful return with some relief and gratitude for getting back on track, but then make some choices. In many cases, we may return to the prior plan without any tending at all to that last moment, the freshly recovered-from pratfall. That's legit; but there are other options to consider.

First, as to that getting back on track: it may be as simple as a knowing return to the object(s) of awareness. As you've likely found in your own budding practice, there's a spectrum of losing attention one way (to a cloud of gnat-like thoughts) or another (a lights-out mental dullness). While I humbly value all aspects of mind as equally worthy, there's a hierarchy in finding our way out of "lost."

When really stuck, resetting at the base of the physical, and especially of the breath, is the most reliable way. A big, deliberate belly breath may be enough, then back out to the plan.

An intermediate intervention is to stay on the breath a bit to reestablish some consistency with keeping attention on a familiar target. Sometimes moving back to the base practice not only rebuilds a little confidence in the moment but creates a brief interlude to watch how mind is being pulled away as it happens in this most familiar practice. "Meta" (watching the quality watching itself) is particularly available for tending to within this basic form.

For a full reboot, the manual here says to hold down the keys H, W, and G. Yes, "HWG" is a go-to start routine, but is also an awesome restart routine: settle in here (wiggling the tush is an effective "Here I am, in the mindscape"); reestablish membership in the Grand Society of the Fellow Mindful-aspiring, as we wrestle with wavicles near and far; and then go back to the intended watching.

Whether or not a full reset or a quick "breather" is the right tool to regain some stability and clarity on the current intention is a matter of some trial and error and incremental learning. Each of us gains insight over time not just of phenomena, but also of our own blind spots and sticking points in meditating and what tools to use in response.

Beyond the reset/restart tactics, a favored tool to reiterate is a checking in with other aspects of the mindscape. For me and a lot of other Western-mind-driven, thought-heavy types, that often involves tending to mental chatter by directing attention into the body and heart—surveying the physical sensation and emotional tone that may be accompanying a runaway narrative going on in OS 3.0 cortex. An intentional, simple "dropping into" shift in attention can truly help, allowing an opening to how (or if) it feels south of the brain.

The slightly more elaborate, imaginal "breathing into" tactic, however comically inflationary in its imagery, is also a trusty tool in keeping awareness below the cranium online. With its rhythmic quality— attention gathered in the in-breath, then directed to the "theme" in the out-breath (followed by an observation of the possible associated qualities)—"breathing into" the moment can provide a structure for holding attention a little more easily.

These tactics can be enough to knock off the repetitive thinking. They also can serve us diagnostically. Stuck spots become demystified by adding in a richer understanding of what that mental moment may be cogenerating physically and emotionally. A surprise may even be found operating in 4.0 as a reduction or increased intensity of meta of the quality of our attending.

These "pattern sets" of OSs—wavicle aspects of body, heart, thought, and awareness, conditioned to emerge together and regularly—become familiar over time. Each of us have our own "greatest hits" of reactive patterns: a portfolio of the most common ones are worth knowing well.

Hack No. 1: Snapshots of the Lost Moment (Before and After)

With developing, skillful application of these tactics to help stabilize fragile moments, the overall confidence in tending to our attentional signal incrementally improves. Wavering attention seems less like "on/off," and more like a dimmer switch. Nevertheless, often attention just drops away with little warning, whether into distracting mental chatter or train-into-a-tunnel dullness. There's that moment of loss, and then one of return; then we may get back on the board, as described. But here's another fruitful option: we can study that lost moment. Let's work backwards.

Instead of either a show trial or a desperate return to home base, right at that sweet spot of regaining awareness, consider a quick step back to observe the return moment itself. Not "judge," but "observe." In that newly resolved loss of awareness might just be evidence of something important that the defensive mind yanked attention away from. So, in coming out of distraction, briefly look around a little bit. Take an extended snapshot of the physical and emotional self; there may be some learning there.

The state of mind just before the lights went out is often harder to recapture. Occasionally a glimpse of something in awareness registers just before the distraction, so it's useful to try to recall to the last remembered "mind event." We can even reset the scene repetitively at the "theme ingredient" and watch what mind does with it in subsequent trials.

Here's another selection on the menu: a "daily special." We will often wrestle with recurring distractions. When working with, say, the breath, is a particular scatter of worrisome thoughts routinely visiting on Sundays, but not Fridays? Does a particular bodily tension between the shoulder blades sting whenever thoughts of an estranged sibling bubble up? Is a heavy heart of gratitude more noticeable when passing by the bakery and its homey smells of goodies?

If a phenomenon or pattern set keeps knocking on the door in the midst of a sitting, you can change things up right then and "turn in" to it. Switch to the new target, not to analyze and add further distraction, but to observe. Running some trials of recurrent observation of the new intruding wavicle of the day can lead to observing what else may be humming underneath, co-occurring, waving at us frantically. As with the other options, consider the "drop into/breath into" maneuver to anchor the "special" distraction to a fuller apprehension of the effect through the OSs.

When nothing's bringing relief from recurrent monkey-mind or slipping into tune out, falling back to the fail-safe tactic of a full reboot is not a white flag of surrender, but a pragmatic, skillful decision. Resettling and wiggling into proper physical position and reiterating the "HWG" or some version of state and plan is a better option than persistent struggle and the additional frustration it can add.

Hack No. 2: Take a Breather...a Quick Mindful Routine

Most meditation guides reinforce the idea that good work put in on the cushion doesn't just generate some benefit during that time of practice, but also develops and cultivates a clearer state of mind off the cushion. And that's true; working in more optimal conditions (a quiet room without interruption, a protected stretch of time) reinforces ways of operating consciously that hopefully become internalized, intuitive, baked-in.

But life mostly happens off the zafu. Intense and/or unexpected events may benefit from a rescue mission or at least a mindful breather. There are dozens of these states that we could work with, but I'll focus on five that I hear about regularly in my work with patients:

- The news, bad or good: a novel moment
- Intense moments: Anxiety and anger
- Craving: alcohol, mood-altering substances, food, digital media, sexy time
- Slothville: Boredom, loss of motivation

We can sketch out a kind of all-purpose, go-to, quick "breather" routine first, then use it to flesh out some variations for the special moments above. First, we'll need to tinker a little with the basic recipe. You remember the basic recipe, right? A setup, then some warm-up breath work to get into a groove, then bring on the intended observation, then wrap up (with an eye on the mind's eye)? Well, as we are tackling moments occurring in less-than-optimal conditions, we'll need to take that into account and simplify things. Three steps here: Setup, Checklist, and Wrap-up. Easy...

The setup: Some bad news about Grandma, or a texting driver weaving into your lane, or a glass of wine offered to a newly-sober you at a party twenty days into recovery: these are not "optimal" settings for settling into a meditative state, however helpful that could be to stabilize body and mind in response. There's no cushion in sight. Yet, with a quick "excuse me for a moment" exit to the restroom or hallway, or even a pulling off of the freeway, we can try to make it work.

The ubiquitous "Here-We-Go" with its built-in three slow breaths can be enough of a launch.

> **"HERE"** embeds the surprising new wavicle in the broader landscape: "Here I am, Chardonnay-craving me on a Tuesday afternoon at the supermarket," for instance. A big belly breath accompanies.
>
> **"WE"** may sound extraneous in the midst of the novel moment, but it can be crucial; "I'm trying to gain some strength here, like, well, most everybody else"—or bring to mind a loved one, family, a congregation, past or present. Never truly alone in this thing; others, somewhere, wrestling with a similar experience. A nice rounded breath, please.
>
> **"GO"** is the intention, usually well-defined: "briefly sit with this $$^&$*&* thing that just happened."

If you only have those three breaths, so be it; if you can take a few more to further set up this first-aid routine, that's even better.

The Checklist: We get out of (just) our heads with this four-step survey. It's a sequential three-stop circuit of observations (physical, emotional, thoughts) and then a fourth step to pull back to an observation of all three together, to observe how the current experience impacts us more completely. Unless the abruptly novel event is a directly physical/sensory one—an athletic injury, a menstrual cramp, an unexpected kiss, etc.[49]—we mostly apprehend a new wavicle in thought, in conceptual recognition. So, a regular directing of attention to the body and heart, and then to the whole, is a brief but more complete tuning into the moment and its impact. So:

- Sequentially attend to the body, heart, and head with at least a mindful breath or two. This is a good pace to use the "breathe into" tactic—inflate away with a sense of tending to the physical state with a couple of breaths, then a recentering on the heart, then up to how the thoughts are perking.

- Finish by pulling back as possible to an observation of all three, awareness filling all of you. Notice how it operates all the way through.

The Wrap-up: The conditions for this brief interior check-in routine being imperfect as they are, regularly scheduled life awaits our wrapping up this brief exercise. As with concluding structured meditation sessions, we can employ the familiar symmetry from our planned practices.

- A quick pull out to a "meta" view is always an option— how's my awareness? with a novel event, it's common to perceive a kind of contraction around the new thing. A quick observational snapshot of that can be instructive, even surprising, and allow for a release.

- Open back out and reorient, letting mind settle back, bookended by reiteration of this brief practice now concluded—there, we, are.

That's the routine for unexpected moments: set up a quick break for focused attention; observe the novel wavicle with your breath as a guide, with an intention to capture the experience in a full-ish way;

---

49   My beloved pooch lying at my feet just released some prodigious canine flatus into my current landscape as I am writing this. "Breathing into," indeed.

rest in that observing mind's eye as you wrap up. Taking some brief notes, whether in mind, a quick voice memo on a smart phone, or some bullet points on tieback of a napkin, can also help capture the moment. But then life moves on.

Speaking of moving on, let's apply this routine to those target moments. The Setup/Checklist/Wrap-Up sequence is our framework; there are some specific aspects of these states that this sequence can help highlight and stabilize.

2.1: Gimme the News

While "The News" here as a target for coping could easily refer to the twenty-four-hour talking heads on cable news and blizzard of posts in our smartphone feeds, I truly mean novel information of all sorts, from the boss' abrupt critique of your PowerPoint, to an ominous result on your blood work, to your smiling child's good grade on a project you completed, er, helped with.

The key aspect of news is, well, it's new! New input—new wavicles, really, coming in hot via our senses—challenge and disrupt the current landscape of our minds. There's an activation that inevitably occurs, whether in a big way, like with a phone call from the hospital about the death of a loved one or with the merest tweak perceived in viewing an emoji on a text.

It's novelty, and with novelty brings a burst of reaction that registers in a particular way for each individual. That's really the case for any bit of news, bad, good or in-between. The antidote to that novelty is familiarity, which is where a predictable, handy routine like this helps. A brief break to take a meditative snapshot of the effect is not always or even usually necessary, but a good tool.

As for some particulars about applying the "mindful breather" routine to news:

SETUP: HWG should play a focal role in this brief routine for managing a new input. That initial anchoring in the regularity of setting, belonging, and intention ("take a brief break to let this news settle in") is familiar and usually comforting. "Here" is usually what is not changed in the moment.

CHECKLIST: Most news these days is received in cognitive, thinky form, in through the eyes and/or ears as printed/written or digital media, or spoken or broadcast messages. But input riffles through the whole of us, and the somatic and emotional reaction to new input should not be ignored. The checklist sequence does that. Be aware, also, that the new input circles back up to the thought-deck for another pass, this time in judgment of that new information: like, dislike, or meh. Notice it all with some directed breaths.

WRAP-UP: Again, some symmetry in closing the quick sequence embeds the new stuff in a familiar way. That meta thing is worth emphasizing here. The quality of our awareness tends to shift with something new. However "open" and more spacious our observing self is just before, we usually contract attention around the new bit of information, and in doing so, are distracted from the prior mental landscape, whether fuller or maybe contracted around another thing. This is a good moment for a quick "how's my attention?" step into that meta view. A "there—we—are" (changed, perhaps, by the new input) ending to the breather allows to put the news in place. That may involve a "pocketing" of the news and a return to the pre-novelty plan. The breather may also have provided enough pause and observation to change plans—but creating a moment for a deliberate rather than impulsive change.

Ok—next, let's apply this "breather" sequence to a duo of intense reactions: anxiety and anger.

2.2: Fear and Loathing: Two (Threatening) Sides of a Coin

Anxiety and anger are built-in evolutionary features of human experience. One makes us bolt out of the road rather than smile in our reflection in the shiny chrome bumper careening straight at us. The other signals that we are, well, being messed with. Both are ancient responses, and valid ones, to perceived threats. As we've covered way back in the book, both biology and early entrainment may screw with the volume knob on the intensity of both "fight" and "flight" (and, to be complete, "freeze") in our contemporary lives of intermittent, but usually not life-threatening threat.

While the felt states often feel diametrically opposed, distorted or inappropriate responses of both the anxious and angry flavors can be attended to with our "Breather" routine.

> **SETUP:** Like any new input, "HWG" anchors a flash of exploding panic or intense grievance in a familiar set of opening steps. For both anxiety and anger, the "We" in HWG plays an important signaling role as an antidote to the self-centered quality of these states and how they contract attention around scared or rageful self. Panic anxiety sufferers will recognize the reflexive "me, all by myself" in that state: "I'm losing control!" The enraged may embrace the "me, the victim" in that state of angry activation, but actually need a quick dose of "We," of what connects to others, in the midst of an intense moment of feeling messed with, of feeling devalued. "Holding this hot potato" is the "Go" intention, either way.

CHECKLIST: Anxiety and anger generate indelible somatic/emotional marks, often states that feel intolerable to hold. That's the "collapse to 1.0" spin that taking a breather like this is meant to soften and provide an alternative to. Including a belly-breathing "diagnostic" scan through how the experience is registering in body and heart allows a moment for fuller understanding of the impact. The time taken in that scan is not just diagnostic, but also therapeutic: it's slowing down the race to blunt actions of fight or flight, unless truly necessary.

WRAP-UP: Building a disciplined interior response to difficult moments like these includes finishing the steps, including the meta, "here's me, holding this state...how's that going?" The immersion in "freaked" or "pissed" shifts to those as an object of awareness for the moment. The breather may have also provided enough pause and observation to change plans—but creating a moment for a deliberate, rather than impulsive change.

2.3: The Pause, You Crave

The ache that comes with dependence on—as well as breaking that dependence from—any number of additives and inputs is a state that can range from a mere whisper to a blaring alarm. How craving as a kind of suffering operates is a complex topic. The constellation of phenomena we recognize as craving is informed by genetics-driven neurochemistry, more in some than in others. Early life entrainment and conditioning reinforces the loop. Of course, exposure to the substance or sensory ticklers in the current moment grossly contribute to the difficulty, as anyone mesmerized by smell of french fry grease or freshly baked cookies can attest to. For others, it's a freshly lit cigarette. The activation of sexual craving has proliferated in the last generation from magazines under the bed to most every form of public media.

Craving as an aspect of the drama of drug addiction gets most of the press in the mass media. Similar neurochemistry also drives the addiction to sugar and carbs. It works in the other direction, too. Mass media ads create sensory triggers of craving: the slo-mo ooze of cheese on the TV burger ad or the inviting sweat on the bottle of beer (not to mention on the curves of the model holding the brew).

Craving drives the virtual world, too. Witness the quick glimpse of the curves on a photoshopped model embedded in an otherwise antiseptic internet article. The ubiquitous "play again?" clicks on video games. Or the noxious goosing up of our political ire on digital platforms—that's a craving too: for the validation and amplification of grievance. Current social media algorithm software, fine-tuning our individual craving preferences to target eyeballs and dollars, certainly does not help.

For those wrestling with the early recovery phase of sobriety from alcohol, narcotics, stimulants, or other drugs, that craving signal registers throughout, regarding of our map. We feel it in the body (restlessness, tremor, a circus in the bowels), heart (anxiety, the fear of relapse, the anticipated shame of that aftermath, and more), and head (a swarm of chatter: Where can I get some? Can I live without it? How will I explain it away?)

All that suffering is an itch that calls out for a scratch, and, for many of us, the stakes are profound. A quick and slippery slope back into complete chemical chaos can ruin a life. For others, it's a broken promise to a loved one to "scale it back" that takes another brick out of the home of matrimony, maybe the one that knocks the house down.

A mindful routine to manage craving is not a substitute for a fully-figured treatment plan to get and stay back in control of whatever

Siren is beckoning. We all can give in to the song. Obviously, there are entire industries devoted to the control of our uncontrolled appetites, featuring programming from Jenny to Betty to Bill W. My intent here is not a simplistic, foolish, "meditate your addiction away!" alternative to addiction treatment, but as an additional tool.

There are those inevitable moments, whether in treatment or not, where craving is an immediate thing, an emergent moment. The blunt goal in managing these momentary blasts of craving is in a bare enduring of the experience without acting on it. The cognitive behavioral therapy books call it "E & RP": exposure and response prevention. As in, with exposure to the experience, prevent a quick "rescue" response; don't scratch the itch, but instead, ride it out, reduce the sensitivity and prove some control. That's a radical kind of adaptation. A plan would be helpful.

We can interpose a brief commercial break in the service of our autonomy of a 4.0, "let's look at craving me," pause for observation and deliberation prior to consequential reaction.

With that brisk introduction into the fraught world of intense "gimme," let's run the routine:

SETUP: The "Here" in HWG can be crucial in managing craving, as it drives some embedding of the longing in the setting around, which may well be a triggering or at least complicating factor in that craving. Let me provide some examples: "here in a hotel bar, ten days into my recovery;" "here with my damn phone pinging texts from my ex while I'm sitting at a stoplight; "here walking through the food court on my way to my job." Here at least opens up a window to the conditions around— perhaps to alter them, but at the least to be informed. While "Here" may be a diagnostic aid, "We" is just as important as a therapeutic step. We can conjure the comfort of one's home twelve-step group, or spiritual clique, or an ideal figure in imagination or history who's wrestled successfully with the craving of the moment. "We" creates a team in mind—"we can do this."

CHECKLIST: Craving involves a wide variety of intensities and characteristics, depending on the kind. In the instance of alcohol, there's a shape to the intensity based in the half-life of alcohol as its ebbs from the body and brain. Many individuals trying to manage the craving for nicotine report a powerful conditioning aspect in terms of a greater ache tied to particular scheduled times, like after meals, or as a reflexive pull when anxiety kicks up. Substance craving has a potent somatic aspect that begs for a "dropping into" to attend to fully. "Digital"/mental craving often brings with it a swarm of "just this once's" and "if I don't now, I'll miss something's." A brief but disciplined, step-wise survey of the craving's registration in body, heart, thought, and attention fully identifies the challenge. One other benefit: craving naturally wavers, varies, has a beginning and an end. Watching that variability helps reinforce that temporary aspect, and taking that moment to survey also is one more moment to let the novelty of "OMG, I need it" to settle into "there's that craving. I got it."

WRAP-UP: Individuals actively working through addictions, dependencies, and the cravings thereof generally are directed not to toss themselves purposely into provocative, triggering settings and circumstances. Short of such self-sabotage, craving phenomena usually kick up inadvertently, while in the midst of some other moment—maybe at rest (the latest in pizza cheese elastic technology presents itself for your halftime watching pleasure on the couch) or in action (squeezing an impromptu coffee grab into an already compressed commute to work). The point is, we don't cure cravings in these moments, but briefly attend, then get back to the plan, or no plan if that was the, uh, plan. A wrap-up step sets that up: "Ok, proceeding with this craving burden, but I'm aware of it better now—let's go."

2.4: Welcome to Slothville

In the vast landscape of our minds' many moments is the often-obscured municipality of...Slothville. In its city limits include the creatures of boredom, lost motivation, inertia, and perceived "laziness," all hanging lazily from trees as we amble through town. They appear to be located on the other side of the tracks of our more active states of our experience. They may not even seem like "states" at all. But they too are moments that we can learn to observe, hold, and adapt to.

I happen to think these experiences are surprisingly under-explored and thus misunderstood. Therapists and patients may ignore them and miss undercurrent anxiety, sadness, or passive rebellion, blanketed over by a too-easily accepted fog of "I'm just that way"— today, or even most every day. Folks I work with are sometimes surprised by my meditative homework assignment between sessions: to treat "bored" or "flat" as a thing to drop into, look at more closely. And another cryptic instruction: that the perceived OS 1.0 fatigue may actually be a 4.0 attentional tune out. However ironic a "breather" routine is to observe what seems like a mind stuck in neutral, that routine can flex to work here.

SETUP: Sometimes the simple pivot to the setting of place, belonging, and intention is enough to help anyone move out of a dull state. "HWG," after all, is a decision, an action with a purpose. Moving through the rest of a brief "breather" routine may become moot as the setup itself drives some get up and go...

and that's just fine. Yet "here, feeling like a sloth," visualizing a society of fellow sloths, and "let's look at my own slothiness for a minute" can shed some light on the details of the experience and the moment it's embedded in or hanging from. So consider finishing the routine out.

CHECKLIST: Inertia can really find its way in any or all of the four realms of experience we check here. But it's most likely that the realm of awareness itself is the lead sloth, dampening any sharper attention paid to what may register in the body, any fog obscuring the emotional weather, or any dullness of thinking. We can particularly use an overall dulling subconsciously and reflexively to mute uncomfortable or noxious states and patterns underneath. Some examples: tending to body sensations can register fatigue, and linked, emotional disappointment in recent weight gain or loss of stamina from a bailed-on workout program. Breathing into the emotional realm may uncover that "blah" is actually defending against some intense grievance that is hard to hold or with no available other to vent it at or to. Checking into "slowed thinking" may reveal, well, slowed thinking (am I getting enough rest? or too much cannabis?), but also could shine an attentional light on some difficult decisions to make, problems to work through, mental challenges that risk failure and resultant shame. In short, boredom and inertia can be defenses against other more active but tough stuff. So we try to breathe through the fog, take a quick peek, and maybe learn something new.

WRAP-UP: I find nothing too special about wrapping this flavor of "breather" routine up, except for noting that it's meant to be a curious investigation into various forms of slowing, not a rigid antidote. Even with a more informed view of "sluggish me," we still have the autonomy to stay at rest, and that may be the right thing to do. The intention here is to know these states, like any other, more fully—with the hunch that there may be more to the sloth than meets the eye.

Some metaphors—ok, clichés—may nevertheless help round out this "breather" routine work. The state of craving (or the other states of discomfort described above), once identified and briefly demystified, can be visualized as, say, a pebble in the shoe. With time pressing to move along, we can choose to notice that pebble but keep walking rather than let it stop us cold. We can attend to the (ouch!) additional wavicle, but not get irrevocably distracted by it. We breathe into the ouch a bit, note its qualities, and walk on.

One other metaphor can help, especially around a mind full of incessant chatter: a business or other group meeting. Most of us have endured the experience of an attendee droning on, repeatedly driving an obvious point home like a toddler pounding a plastic hammer on that round peg, perhaps into a square hole. The secret sauce of a brief "dropping into" a tough state is that in that action we also drop back, back to observation, resting back home in the meta/watcher mode.

The pitch here to whatever uncomfortable phenomenon of experience is driving the tension: give it a seat at the table, listen briefly, but you run the meeting.

Hack No. 3: Mindful Bracketing

While most of us benefit from setting a routine time for daily practice, whether mornings, or evenings, or sometimes both, life usually happens in between. We've been covering the unexpected occurrences that can rattle us, surprise us, and perhaps change us in fruitful ways, if we are able to apply some attentional effort. The "breather" routine can become second nature over time and practice:

when something novel happens, we can skillfully take a quick gander at the effect on the mindscape.

Other life events are less immediate, more predictable, and can be enhanced in awareness by a slight variation on this brief, mindful practice. It's not, "Seven o'clock and time to sit." Nor is it, "a pink slip? Right now? I need a (mindful) breather." This practice is something in between: a routine but brief opener and closer to the daily actions and activities that many of us engage in but can sometimes lose the energy, intention, and appreciation for in the midst of a blur of contemporary life. Think of it as the mindful theme song[50] to your own show: play it to lead you to a defined stretch of action, and then play it back out.

What kinds of action? I've found recommending this bracketing routine helpful for individual workdays, whatever the jobs—but especially ones that involve direct tending to others. Teachers dig it as a brief interlude to set their mind and intention straight prior to the scramble of kids flooding the classroom, and then later on after the room empties. I've employed the same tactic in teaching bigger kids—a brief tune in before lecturing to training docs, then a quiet check-in moment after I've covered the last PowerPoint slide and answered their final questions. Performers—actors, musicians, dancers, creatives of all stripes—can bracket their performances in this way. Newbie self-help book authors find that bracketing my, um, their writing sessions helps to identify and settle tension, and then guide awareness in a productive direction. Or so I hear.

It is a vital, essential moment in my own clinical workday. Even if I only have a minute, I prep for my first patient of the day with a brief, planned opening in compassionate awareness. At the end of

---

50   "Who lives in a pineapple under the sea?" Taken. As is "I'll be There for You" by The Rembrandts. Be your own one-hit wonder!

my workday, I try to bookend that brief meditation with a closing snapshot of, "done...how did that impact me?"

I can't with any certainty claim invention or discovery of this "hack" highlighting the entries and exits from personal efforts, though I haven't seen it specifically elaborated on much elsewhere. My own happening upon this routine came by accident, by desperation, really, in returning to clinical practice after radiation treatment and some complications thereof. With the intense distractions of somatic side effects of the treatment and a boatload of steroids aboard to treat those lovely effects, I found myself pretty damn immersed in suffering self. A Michelin Man morphing of body, a hair-trigger irritability of heart, and brittle distractibility of my ol' reliable thinky brain greeted me each morning as I opened up shop with the aspiration to attend to others and their suffering.

Our own suffering makes us contract our awareness around the aching self. But my particular job, not so unlike any other job that requires full attention to another individual, relies on opening out, not contracting in. Grunting through, or even tuning out, my own difficult stuff would also be quite the mixed message conveyed to my patients—folks I've routinely urged to bravely tune in to their own difficult stuff. It'd be a denial of the obvious, some ripe hypocrisy in action. Yet rather than switching chairs and leaking all over people counting on me to help them, I recognized the need for cultivating a middle ground: holding my own tension, even modeling the managing of it, in a way that allowed me to be effective in the interaction.

A mindful check-in of state, belonging, and intention (that's HWG) bloomed out of that brainstorming for a "play-in theme" sufficient to cultivate that necessary state of mind. Yeah, that damned thing again. Nothing fancy here; we'll just recycle the ol' H, W, and G, with a couple of emphases.

- The "Here" noting of self, state, and setting pulls us into the scene, whether it's prior to walking on stage, or "my date will be here in five," or anticipating an interview, or the rush of a family in weekday evening flux (homework, dinner, bedtime battles, etc.)

- The "We" step may seem unusual to include as a regular aspect of prepping for action, but I actually think it's essential and workable in a couple of ways. One is in visualizing other peers in the task, all humbly managing our parallel experiences somewhere, somehow. For me, maybe it's a shared bond of shrinks laboring at our work; perhaps we can get a group discount on tissues. Or "We" can cast a broader net to fellow wavicles at the service of others. That's some union.

- Another flavor of "We" to consider embracing is the "We" of the other party or parties in the interaction(s) to come, whether that be with the patients in the waiting room, the audience silencing their cell phones, or the prospective caller to the support phone line one is preparing to manage (this last one helps me personally when I'm dialing an insurance company about a messed-up claim). Except in rare cases of overt prepping for battle, most of our interactions in the day-to-day involve at least the option of bonding, of creating a positive alliance, of empathy and compassion. Bringing to mind the opportunity for "We," for a bond of belonging, doesn't mean dropping one's reasonable defenses nor a foolish "kick me" vulnerability. But humans are more hardwired by nature for threat, less so for "win-win." This step helps counter that.

- The "Go" is straightforward—with the landscape attended to and a nod to our coming partner(s) in the dance, we go. Simple enough, but note how many times each of us sleep-walks into a task, relying on intuition and repetition to launch, and without a discrete intention in mind. As with sitting meditation, this "Go" step reinforces awareness of a deliberate effort to be made. It defends against the half-assed effort. Put the whole behind in there.

Speaking of halves, the other half of this bracketing routine is meant to close out the action with attention to registering the event's impact on one's current state, and reiteration of connection, and a proper closing. "TWA" is another familiar recycling project; here are a few pointers.

"THERE" is really "here," in terms of a similar, brief survey of the state of body, heart, head, and looker. But consider how often we complete or perhaps endure a planned event or action, then barrel ahead to the next one without any attempt to let the last one sink in. Even a directed few breaths to center the self and take stock can be instructive, if only to pause for a decision about how/whether to proceed to the next thing. And that pause can refresh, as the old cola ad reminds us.

"WE" is still "we"—a quick nod or even goodbye to the dance partner of the completed task or event. It can be a reinforcement of the imaginal posse of fellow craftspeople. It can even be a pivot to a broader "we"— to one's own family to return to at the end of a hard day, or the broadest "we" of fellow wavicles striving for some contentment. We still belong, even after the dance.

"ARE" puts a deliberate period at the end of the sentence, an intention to shift from going to being, from action to rest. Again, this may seem simple in understanding, but routinely ignored for many of us in our sequenced, busy life schedules. We don't truly

separate from the last task, especially in judgment of the thing and our role. Thinking about the last event, critiquing and analyzing is inevitable; "thought stopping" about this or anything else is an oxymoron. But an intentional nod to "done" can help move us out of that loop of chatter and back to a meta space—"me, observing myself at rest." Even if it is a restless rest.

A perhaps cliché but nevertheless true statement is that anything and anytime can an opportunity for mindful observation. The converse holds, too: any moment can be lost to mindlessness. Most are, actually. But we can set some fruitful conditions by these intention-setting brackets for planned activities—HWG in, TWA out.

Let me close this chapter with an example of successful use of the "mindful breather" tactic in a tragi-comic vignette. It comes from my own recent surgical history. You may wish to read it aloud, perhaps with an ominous Anthony Hopkins accent for effect.

I'll Share: (No) Silence of the Lambs

In early 2012, an MRI of my neck region delivered me some dreadful news: that my malignant chondrosarcoma was back in business, growing again. It had been a mere fourteen months after I'd had neurosurgery to mostly excavate the little bastard of a malignant tumor torturing my poor plexus of nerve roots running out from my spinal cord to keep the lights on in my left shoulder and arm. The new input generated a mix of intense reactions for me to handle.

One was deep threat. Research I'd done into the possible trajectories of recurrence of my flavor of cancer suggested that while whacking it back can sometimes scare the thing into remission, the more likely and ominous scenario was of a tumor that accelerates its pace—the cells getting more pathologic in look under the microscope and the tumor more aggressive in its expansion. So, a shudder there in terms of what to do to try to stop the freight train.

Another was, frankly, confusion. I didn't feel like I had "it" again. The initial tumor had truly jacked up my suffering with a chronic, worsening dull ache and explosions of intense pain that often ripped me out of sleep. After the surgery and up to the evidence of recurrence, I was gratefully free of the worst of that mess. There'd been no uptick in symptoms post-surgery, so the new bomb was ticking pretty quietly.

Ultimately, a grim kind of acceptance set in that I was in for a long, maybe unending stretch of battle and uncertainty. I got seconds and thirds opinion-wise on next steps, then settled back with my ace surgeon with the direction to whack the tumor back further but try to preserve function in my dominant left arm and hand. When I awoke in the recovery room from surgery, I faced a truly novel moment, one that one can prepare only so much for, mindfulness or not: does it still work? Tears came to my eyes as I lifted my arm and wiggled my fingers like a baby. My beloved was sitting at my bedside, and seemed less thrilled than I, which was a little weird. She looked like she needed to tell me something.

Just then, a different kind of novelty. My surgeon walked in and delivered the radical news that my wife had been about to drop on me (my brave spouse!) The surgery plan of the day had been scrapped early on, as when opened me up he found another, much larger hunk of tumor, poorly visualized on the MRI (nothing's perfect) but wrapping around my spinal cord. So instead of the targeted trim of the growth out the side of my spine (just a little off the side, please), he gamely switched gears and took out the riskier hunk of badness and most of the vertebra it was attached to. I was now the proud owner of a titanium vertebral body, and a plate, and some rods and screws to hold it all together. A Home Depot of a neck.

(And an amazing, courageous job by my surgeon, to whom I'm eternally grateful.)

As I absorbed that news, still wiggling my fingers, the capper was that all that emergent work took so much time and effort that going after the original growth had to be scrapped that day. My hand worked because its function hadn't been threatened (yet). And I'd be coming back in a week or so for Round Two.

I can't say I "decided then and there to apply the Mindful Breather© tactic, with its customary effectiveness," as much as it occurred to me that in the shock of all that input, those interesting, unprecedented conditions, I sort of intuitively fell back on a simple checklist of observation. I'd been prepping prior to surgery to fall back on whatever I knew to help in metabolizing the "expected" variables in outcome. But this was even outside of what I'd anticipated. More orthodox meditating would follow, but in a bed with lines and tubes Gulliver-ing me in place and a tinker toy neck encased in a brace, a checklist to "breathe" through my experience in body (ow!), heart (OMG!), head (WTF!), and watcher (a bit dulled by both events and pain meds) was a welcome plan to get me through the next hours.

I introduced this vignette as "tragi-comic," and some readers may be wondering about my sense of humor. I'll finish this tale with another moment I had to breathe through, lest "Murder in the Neuro Ward" would have graced the newspaper the following day. After a mere few hours in the ICU as a precaution, I was told I was stable enough for transfer to room on the main floor, but that as the hospital was crowded, the bed would be in the neurology unit, which on that evening featured a number of unfortunate, neurologically confused patients prone to wandering.

Hospital policies have evolved for good clinical and legal reasons to frown on tying people down to their beds in these circumstances. Instead, the unit employed what I suppose were considered "cheerful" alarm systems on the beds of the intrepid wanderers, sounding whenever there was an attempted escape. Each alarm itself played an electronic version of the children's classic, "Mary Had A Little Lamb," in sonic tones that roughly resembled an ice cream truck's broadcast. It was bahhhhd.

There were four wanderers. So, four alarms. Maybe five. Turned up loud. Deep into the night. Not in unison (the wanderers should have eloped en masse, but it was not to be). Occasionally the versions would line up, or sound like a "Frère Jacques"-style round. But mostly, it was a phenomenon that the CIA should really consider.

The understaffed and overmatched nurses and aides couldn't keep up. I rang once when a particular alarm had not been tended to for what seemed like hours, to ask for relief from the sound as well as a little extra pain medicine and the hope for blessed unconsciousness in the midst of pre-school-flavored acoustic torture.

Otherwise, it was another moment for a "mindful breather"—at first as a ritual distraction from the noise, then just a "spot" treatment when the symphony would become especially raucous. The wanderers and their sonic flock eventually tired and knocked out, as did I. (I begged for discharge the next morning.)

To wrap the tale up: I had the following ten days to pull things together and heal a little, then back in for the second surgery. Another recovery room moment of intense novelty, my sweetie by my side. I groggily awoke, wiggled my fingers…my ace surgeon had done it again! Tears in my eyes, then, I nodded off.

Then, a different kind of goofiness. If you've ever had surgery, or even a procedure such as an endoscopy or colonoscopy, you may be familiar with the effect of a particular medication in the mix. It's an effective short-acting sedative yet has unusual effects on memory. For some, it can impact any memories that occurred not only just after its administration ("anterograde amnesia"), but for events occurring minutes prior ("retrograde amnesia"). In some past surgeries, I'd woken up with some irritable commentary along the lines of "let's get this show on the road, what are we waiting for?" requiring my remarkably patient sweetie to remind me that the surgery had been completed already. And again, when I'd fall asleep briefly, then wake to harangue anyone in earshot about said show and the awaiting road. For my poor wife, a kind of anesthetic Groundhog Day of anterograde amnesia to help me through.

With this surgery, though, I exhibited the marvel of retrograde amnesia and a broken record of the Hallmark card moment. I'd wake, register deep joy and gratitude at my good fortune of surviving intact, then nod off. And again. Take three. Take four. I eventually stayed awake with a sustained sense of gratitude.

Into the Deep End

Hopefully you are gaining some confidence in the practice of meditation and some appreciation of its benefits, including the use of the tactics involved. In addition to the regular practice, we can apply the tools of the trade in tight spots of momentary novelty, difficult and acute states, and as a mindful "before/after" framing of events.

We've covered a fairly thorough survey of the landscape of individual "constructed" self, the perspective we most always hold in navigating the day to day of our lives. We drew some maps, then started with the "home base" of our observed breath, in and out. It made sense to use that base to build some comfort, if not mastery, the basics of observing, the losing and regaining, and the sneak-peaks of experience we can sometimes get just before we get lost in dullness or distraction. Hopefully, a developing tolerance for the inevitable ups and downs of the work, as well as some budding sense of benefit, has also grown out of that wheezing training camp.

Part II's practices were meant to build on that foundation and open up practice to the wider extent of our "layered" selves—to the full "soma," then to emotional "weather fronts," and up to the range of ways mind produces and amplifies thoughts. Through all, the emphasis has been on an ongoing cultivating of the "watcher," the observing you that is always present, even when the other wavicles in the scene come and go. I've stressed that *"meta"* quality, of observing your own awareness itself for clarity, for spaciousness versus tight contraction and states in between. We've worked little by little on that essential but underappreciated key of the meditating process all through the preceding practices.

The last part of the book is meant to give an entry-level glimpse into the opportunity for attending to the big-M field itself, beyond yet in the midst of the critters roaming the landscape, the coming and going wavicles of the moment. In the big picture, those phenomena are the observations of little-m mind, immersed in big-M. So now we head into that deep end with some practices designed for creating the opportunity for witnessing deeper states.

This entry may seem to some a step beyond "beginners' training"— not practical in a book harping on practicality. Yet for many, these deeper states of awareness can and do emerge unbidden off the cushion—on a walk in nature, in a structured spiritual setting, or in the midst of some other moment. In the process of the valuable, more stress management-based work of the rest of *Practical Mindfulness,* you may have already had such moments, whether as a whisper or a shout. It's only sensible to have some familiarity with what others have commonly observed of this experience. There are some particular qualities to attend to that we'll explore.

And, it must be stressed (hah!) that "chasing" after tastes of the nondual is neither practical nor particularly effective. Like the other work we've done, it's another example of setting ourselves up in an optimal state for observation—with curiosity and some humility. We run the exercise and witness what happens.

PART III

CHAPTER 13

It's All Home:
Deeper Awareness

The final sets of practices in *Practical Mindfulness* will structure routines for observing the, um, structureless.

Observe what, now? Is that really practical?

You may remember back in the first few chapters that I framed out a conceptual big picture, that what each of us operate in, in the day-to-day living of lives, is our construction of a separate self. It's not "fiction," at least in my view of it, but our sense of an individually aware self is a necessary "home" we build atop what quantum physics has proved is one endless field of energy, flowing and connected—what I've short-handed as "Vibe." The complex science behind how that energy—capable of both flowing like waves and becoming "bound" in form, in particles, in matter—operates, well, that's beyond my pay grade. But it does lead to the opportunity to pursue what aspect of our felt state of momentary experience is our construction, and what might be that undercurrent connection, available for our perception.

The "maps" and practices so far in *Practical Mindfulness* have focused on developing and training up the basic capacity of mindful attention. Through attending to an aspect of experience—the breath, an emotion, a pattern of thoughts recurring—we practice to gain a deepening familiarity with this attention capacity as its own valuable thing to know well, and ultimately to rest in as the "home" of mind.

With the over-and-over resetting, losing and regaining of that awareness, and applying to any and every wavicle in our perceived fields, we each build stretches of more clarity in each moment of the observing and the ability to sustain those stretches without losing attention as easily.

We also have a long lesson in humility and frustration tolerance as the wild wavicles of the field drag our attending selves off routinely into mindlessness. Some days are worse than others, regardless of the practice. Practicing with a variety of wavicles to "work with," whether of our choice, or with whatever arises in that particular moment, we start to cultivate a leave-the-judgment-at-the-door patience for whatever we get that day, on the cushion and especially off. We also start to develop our own familiarity with the particular stuff of our experience that is more likely to generate dissonance inside, emotional reactions, and a loss of our calm, abiding awareness—yes, also on and off the cushion. Especially off.

I'll reiterate that ironic point that even tough days in meditation, with lots of struggle to maintain a simple watching of wheezing, can be really valuable in a "what keeps pulling me away?" way. It's all good.

If you've been practicing along, you know by now—it's not easy. But it's fruitful in knowing the home of mind well, in understanding, coping with, and managing its distractions. That's a grand benefit all its own and my main goal for you in *Practical Mindfulness*. Yet that work also allows us to perhaps dip a toe into the deeper cosmic pool.

That's this last piece of training: attention on opening to the big-M, that Vibe, the broadest field of quantum energy that all wavicle phenomena are built from and immersed in and that we commonly lose sight of amid our constructed lives and their distracting patterns. That cosmic backdrop, and its observation from true landscape view, can be the ultimate setting for a practice.

We have plenty of time and space around the bend[51] to take a look at deeper awareness skills and start training them up. But first, a little refresher on that little-m/big-M dilemma is in order.

A Little History (I'll Bring the Schnitzel)

It's not new, this tussle about explaining reality as rooted only in separate, individual experiences—"dualistic" is the philosophical jargon—versus also in a deeper, shared, "nondual" space. Most Eastern wisdom traditions have contended, in their various flavors, that existence is ultimately one endless whole of belonging, an undercurrent state that has been concluded in part through multitudes of individuals perceiving direct, deeper experiences that are distinctly different from the day-to-day "feel" of "me," the individual. But measurable proof of a deeper reality, of a broadest field of energy, has only come courtesy of the more recent findings of quantum physics.

The genius pocket-protector types that developed the quantum framework wrestled with the obvious comparisons that one can make between a scientifically informed "field of energy" and a spiritually or philosophically contended "field of cosmic consciousness." The scientific bigshots of the period, including Heisenberg, Niels Bohr, Wolfgang Pauli, Ernest Schrödinger, and the OG himself, Albert Einstein, debated how to square up this new reality of quantum to accommodate the perceived reality of the individual observer and his or her impact. Bohr was a big fan of Baruch Spinoza, the humble seventeenth century lens grinder/philosopher, who famously framed matter and mind as "complementary aspects of an ultimate nature." Ultimately, most of the quantum superfriends developed variable

---

51   Quantum joke...killed at the physics conference stand-up night.

spins on the conundrum of mind and matter, if not proclaiming any great certainty about them.[52]

From the Enlightenment on, most Western philosophical and scientific thought has centered on the individual mind as the sole (or, for some, "soul") unit that perceives reality and observes experiences. Whether we approach the topic of experience from a psychological or a biological "mindset," the backstory assumption is of an individual self with a corresponding "mind," "set" in the brain and physically separate from the world to be perceived. There's a self, and the rest... not-self.

From this angle, we can identify a more recent split in investigation, one down the road of orthodox psychoanalytic study of the little-m mind, the other more biological and neurochemical. I alluded earlier to this psychology/biology scrap generating a parallel tussle in modes of treatment as I personally experienced in contemporary psychiatric training. Sigmund Freud, ironically trained as a neurologist, developed and formulated the core elements of a metaphoric framing of how the mind does its thing, starting with the major innovation of categorizing an individual's psychic structure as a conscious part and another part "under that." We've come to accept that the individual mind has its conscious and aware aspects in awake consciousness, but that much of what we experience slips under the waves of awareness to an un-, or subconscious[53] aspect of mind—a mystery component, one that operates and modifies our view of things as we lay down more history with subsequent experience and contemplation.

Freud developed an additional metaphoric way of identifying aspects of mind: the scrabbling trio of id, ego, and superego. The power/

---

52   Heisenberg undoubtedly was most "uncertain" about wearing his superfriends cape. And maybe his briefs on the outside of his leotard.

53   Psychoanalysts can get their sweater-vests in a bunch over the particularities of these basically interchangeable terms. Look out when we start pulling on each other's little goatees.

impulse/pleasure-hungry id and nagging/scolding/do-gooder superego can be simplistically viewed as the mind's Goofus and Gallant,[54] with the ego an orchestrating but impressionable "self" trying to make sense of the other two battling siblings. Lots of breath and ink have been expended, and perhaps boxes of tissue hurled, in arguing over the precise meanings of these metaphoric constructs. But my emphasis here is of the mind as an individual, little-m entity only, and the fruition of an individual brain. Freud's protégé-turned-frenemy, Carl Jung, moved ultimately out of the "little-m mind only" lane, speculating on mind as both an individual entity but also carrying patterns and information of a holistic, collective body of experience and history.

In the last fifty years, neurobiologists have understandably hogged most of the press. Remarkable tools in imaging anatomic byways and corners of the brain have been developed, and molecular discoveries in modifying and manipulating cascades of neurotransmitters have utterly transformed the biological approach to psychiatric suffering.

These momentous developments also the individual mind as the target for the most part. But first, we should try to find it.

(I can imagine Heisenberg, palm to forehead: "Ich habe das schon mal gehort."[55])

I Lost My Mind (or Can't Really Find It to Begin With)

The separate vs. connected conundrum is also reflected in the dustup over the "where" of mind. Pinning down the location of anyone's mind as a discrete functional place is elusive. Millions of hopeful, then hope-dashed meditators have sat with the old Buddhist

---

54 Highlights for Children reference…OK, Boomer!
55 "I've heard this one before."

contemplative practice of first settling one's mind into observing the landscape of stuff in awareness, then being directed to "look for what is watching it all." Much desperate striving and grasping at thin air ensues. It is irritably difficult to locate, at least in physical space. There's no "there" there.

But, you say, there is so much medical evidence that the brain is the physical manifestation of mind, right? After all, if I run my head into a wall, my brain suffers measurably; check the PET scan, the MRI, and the EEG. Memories—a function of mind, we'd mostly all agree on—can get altered too. Isn't that a chunk of brain function gone, ergo, that's mind?

The hair-splitting here is whether brain generates mind, or instead reflects, or even picks up the "signal" of mind. We seem to easily accept, with circumstantial evidence, that something physical, namely our neurological apparatus, creates something completely nonphysical: the experience of mind.

This reductive view seems to frame mind as taking place only inside the noggin. It insists that if brain is associated with mind, it must solely make mind, must generate mind. As a metaphor, if the TV is turned off, one's observation of the big game goes black, but we don't take this interruption in our awareness to mean that the players all stopped playing, then hit the showers and their Twitter feeds.[56]

Taken to its irrational extreme by hard-core neuroscientists, mind gets framed as a mere side effect of the brain. It's cultivated a clinical outlook that insists that if a medication can influence brain chemistry, then mental disorders—in a true sense, suffering associated with awareness—are solely matters of brain chemistry.

Yet, biologists are coming around in the search for experiences of the nondual. Research started in the '60s on the use of psychedelic and

---

56　#confoundingexistentialquestion.

profoundly mood-altering substances (primarily LSD, the psilocybin mushroom, MDMA, and ketamine) to access, or perhaps mimic, states of experience that have been described by meditative adepts. As well-described in Michael Pollan's excellent, recent history of that research, *How to Change Your Mind*, that research got deep-sixed in the '70s as collateral damage of the emerging "War on Drugs." But it's making a comeback in the last fifteen as we try to find relief for those with intractable suffering from depression, anxiety, and especially PTSD. There is interesting work in understanding empathic reactions via "mirror neurons" and subtle energy fields.

As another recent convener of ideas East and West, the physicist and author Fritjof Capra built on Bohr's work, "...trying to harmonize our position as spectators and actors in the great drama of existence." Capra's 1975 book *The Tao of Physics* gets deeply into the interesting weeds of connections between quantum physics and Eastern mysticism and is worth digging into for curiosity's sake. But there it is, again and again: trying to suss out being both watcher and player, observer and immersed, mind and matter. Not either, but both. Wavicles.

To wear out the prevailing metaphor of the book, we're engaging the prospect that our "home" is everywhere. "I'm home" has an endless connotation beyond the keys to the front door and beyond the self we live in and identify with.

The question beckons: can we observe that aspect of experience? What's it like? How can we tell? This last set of exercises offers some opportunities to open to that by first identifying some qualities that have animated the descriptions of the many who have written about it. Then we'll engage some last practices that offer some possibilities.

CHAPTER 14

Into the Deep End: Vibe Practices

While I enjoy watching sports on television, the post-
game interviews can be harder to watch. A particular pet peeve
for me is the ubiquitous, "so, what was that like for you, when you
[dunked it over a seven-footer, hit a hundred m.p.h. fastball out of
the park, threaded the needle between three defenders for game-
winning touchdown pass, etc.]?" Yeah, what *was* that like for you?
The question seems lazy, the answer usually following suit.

Yet sharing these interior experiences of the dropping away of the
patterning of conventional self and the experiencing of something
different and more profound, that's a valid query. There's no field level
camera or instant replay to make an examination of the purported
"unity" experience of big-M any easier. But we do have two-plus
millennia of individual reports to draw upon with some common
themes that emerge.

Also, among some there's also this weird taboo about sharing
individual meditative experiences, especially of this type. These
experiences are admittedly hard to describe and prone to being
misunderstood. Some meditators may defend against their own
acceptance of such contemplative states by dismissing theirs or others'
as fantasy. Many have a rule-bound sense of pristine privacy around
the experience, at least outside of a retreat or teaching/consulting
setting, much like the psychotherapy deal regarding sensitive private

information. In these ways and others, what may be a profound moment can be a minefield to explore in community.

But that shouldn't stop us. We can go there. So...what is that like for you?

From a cosmos full of variations and despite those obstacles, many interior spelunkers[57] through the ages have in fact bravely shared their own explorations. I've researched many of those testimonies, surveyed a mess of individual reports from fellow meditators, and of course examined my own experiences, looking for intersubjective similarities of reported qualities.

Like usual, my goal here is to herd all of these various wavicle cats toward a user-friendly and memorable summary. In service of keeping your attention, I've boiled the critical attributes down to a mere threesome.

The BFB[58]

I distinguish these three aspects as most commonly reported in experience of the "oceanic" or "unity" thing:

- 🍥 a feeling of *expansiveness*
- 🍥 a perception of the *easing away of a sense of separate self* in both space and time, those boundaries feeling less solid and *more fuzzy*
- 🍥 despite that relaxing of a grip on a sense of separate self, a perception of deep *belonging* to the bigness

---

57   Not always a dark night in the soul.

58   With apologies to the estate of Roald Dahl's BFG. The unity experience can indeed even be a BFD.

There are other felt aspects of Vibe discerned, but the big three to observe for skew to a "big/fuzzy/ belonging" (BFB)[59] state. Let's take them one by one.

First, it's big—an expansive, full feeling, with a perceived sense of spaciousness of the field of mind. When we allow details of the pattern sets to be present but do not hyper-focus on them, we may apprehend a more open sense of the field around the stuff we usually dwell on. It's usually a remarkable state to apprehend, at least at first. But it's not necessarily a positive one—more on that in a moment or two.

The Buddhist scholar B. Allan Wallace relates that many report an initial feeling of heaviness atop the head, a washing over the body of energy, and a sensation of "pliancy," of physical lightness and looseness. It's also not unusual to hear reports of alterations in vision and other perception associated with that sense of all-encompassing feeling. Dr. James Austin goes into great detail on the neurologic explanations and speculations that correlate with these felt states. Regardless, one can understand where Freud's favored term "oceanic" comes from. It's what the Buddhists confoundedly often refer to as "emptiness," yet for most it doesn't feel "empty" but instead more "full" and special.

So, "Big." We can sense bigness of the mindscape, keep a look out for its presence.

Next, there is a common sense of "fuzziness" of the borders of self. This may be the hardest to understand and describe. Clearly, one usually perceives where, say, one's backside stops and the chair starts. But what if "my mind" and "this space" is relaxed a bit, even momentarily? The felt state of little-m being immersed in something fuller and bigger—big-M, I've been calling it—opens up. That blurring extends beyond space to a sense of altered time also.

---

59   And you thought we were through with acronyms?

Individuals variously report feel it slowing down or speeding up. In the midst of such immersion experiences occurring during timed sitting periods in meditation, one may feel a half-hour that seemed like an hour or two or, alternatively, just a brief moment.

James Austin refers to the conundrum of "no ready frame of reference" to describe an event which suddenly evaporates or at least loosens the sense of usual, separate physical self in normal time to a "watcher-less," timeless awareness. It is hard to put boundaries and definitions on something defined as a boundary-less state of "no definition," as that would imply a defining quality. But it's a defining component for many, so an identifier is in order.

So, big and fuzzy. The fuzz factor is admittedly a little less identifiable than "big" perhaps, but indelible once you "get" it. We can look for the sense of little-m self getting fuzzy.

A sense of self dropping away could sound freaky, alienating, even deadly in terms of a loss of a personal sense of humanity. Yet, this third aspect is routinely experienced as a warm, benign feeling of belonging, a presence of unity rather than an absence of self. Moreover, it is often identified as positivity itself, a self-less experience of goodness, contentment, and love in a cosmic sense. "Bliss" is a hackneyed but familiar punchline for it.

So, it's a big, fuzzy shift in mind that feels like a hug of belonging. It's BFB.

As an aside, shortly after my own research and summarizing of these "big three" aspects of the deep dive into big-M, and feeling quite proud of myself, I came across the writings of early twentieth century theologian Rudolph Otto who explored what he called the "numinous" state—a term that connotes a deeply felt spiritual experience. He famously distinguished three prime qualities: "tremendum" (call that "big"), "mysterium" (call that "fuzzy"), and "fascinans" (considered to mean potently charming and attractive—

sounds like big-B "belonging.") Of course, Rudolph got there first, as did countless others, no doubt, but it's gratifying to find the similitude.

What happens to our "meta," our individual capacity of awareness? What happens to 4.0 when the other OS's quiet down? Where does our "watcher" go? A common report is a sense of the "me" apprehending BFB loosening, if not outright dissolving, for moments as BFB emerges. This co-occurrence is also a clue toward the little cliffhanger I've hinted at since the early chapters: that the "watcher"—our observing capacity—is also a construction of little-m mind.

Remembering our trusty graphic with puzzle pieces, a field, and a well-manicured eyeball? In fact, it's not just a construction, but the pre-eminent construction of self. This observer is the manufactured entity of our mind we identify with the most. "I'm aware, therefore I am" may need some re-editing.

Here's a try: "I frame a 'little-m me' that's aware, but know it's my own construction of the big-M." That wouldn't fit on a bumper sticker, but there it is.

When we allow for awareness to ease off the familiar distinguishing of "field versus watcher," we can become aware of a continuity, if not a merging at times, of field and watcher. We can rest in the lovely weirdness of just a "watching." Observer and observed, all one thing when we drop back into the big-M.

Just Dropping In

I think of these upcoming practices as approaching the deeper current by "dropping in" or through the distractors that we've become more aware of through our work to date. We attend here preferentially not to the "stuff," but more to the space around the stuff from a couple of different angles: "what else is there, besides these obvious wavicles?" What is it all resting in?

We'll shake the shiny keys of our separate-self phenomena of the field, then yank them away and try to take stock of the mind space that remains. We'll review an ancient technique akin to *Where's Waldo* (or at least the source of his awareness). I'll advance one of my own contemporary spins on these practices that has helped me—a tactic borrowed and adapted from another very old-school exercise in pairing breath meditation to this "little-m meets big-M" aspiration.

In each of these variations, we'll observe the effect on awareness, especially tuning in for the "big three" (BFB) aspects—an expansiveness, a "fuzzy" softening of a self-bound sense of space and time, and a sense of deeper belonging and unity.

Prior to diving in, it's caveat time.[60] Something special in experience sometimes emerges in working with these practices—a shift, a kind of deepening of the moment. And sometimes not. Mostly not, at least early in the game. More than ever, attempting to "force" an outcome usually dooms the exercise. We can set some optimal conditions, then let the moment unfold and try to apprehend, comprehend, and accept whatever occurs subsequently.

Linus in his pumpkin patch may come to mind again, waiting so patiently and then ultimately losing his cool over his, um, squashed hopes for a great visitation. That's an unfortunate but at times apt picture as his subsequent tantrum reflects how it can feel to settle, hold to a dull murmur the chatter of momentary mind, "open out," but then observe...nothing much. Of course, the tantrum is understandable grievance, yet it only "contaminates" the open field a little more. Like so many other lessons in this work, managing that dynamic can become its own beneficial practice.

---

60   As in, "your cosmic mileage may differ..."

That Recipe (With a Few New Spices)

While I have faith that you've been practicing the preceding meditation exercises in all of their glorious varieties, a reminder of that basic sitting routine can't hurt. As with the other practices, it's a meditative sandwich of introductory and concluding steps with the filling of work[61] involving a theme or themes.

> **HWG:** Here (the field), We (not alone), Go (with the intention of engaging a "vibe" practice).
>
> **WARM-UP/META:** Basic watching/losing/regaining attention, starting with breath and moving to a fuller check (body, chakra scan, etc.) of what pattern sets may be "active" in the field; then move attention to the "meta" observing the clarity of awareness itself; that being stable, then...
>
> **MAIN EVENT:** "Vibe" exercises, as will be elaborated on, generally predicated on "what else?"; with those parallel paths of awareness of field with its flow of phenomena, and what happens to awareness in that observation. Ok to get lost, reset, restart; with breaks back on the breath and resettling, then opening back out.
>
> **COOL DOWN:** A move back to a letting go of any direction of awareness, while keeping a "meta" eye on the action...
>
> **TWA:** There (mindscape), We (fellow wavicles), Are (awake and aware as life proceeds).

I've tweaked the recipe a little around the warming up aspect. In most of our practices, our "warming up" stuck close to the breath as the anchor for honing the basic work of holding, losing, and regaining attention. We expanded the warm-up to opening out to landscape

---

61   Even observing baloney and cheese can be nourishing.

view, aiming to build facility in shifting our awareness from "in close" to "way out" and back.

For this ultimate routine, we shift our intention from the careful pattern-set observation to a broader opening—an "outside-in" view of the field, stuff and all, and its qualities as a big-M whole. Hopefully, our conditioned reactions and counteractions are becoming more familiar and identifiable. So, we can build that observation into the warm-up—a "warm-up plus" that includes a cursory "pattern-set scan," though those sets will likely pop up and we will notice them as we proceed with our sequential warm-up observations. With some stability and clarity in attention cultivated over, say, five to ten minutes, the turbo warm-up concludes with moving out to the widest angle, to "meta"—watching it all, including attending to the clarity of the watching.

Knowing one's own patterning well is a premium here, as getting intensely caught up in the sensation, emotion, narrative, and/or shift in awareness driven by any prominent presence in momentary mind makes this next task, an opening to, "what else, besides that stuff," a tougher one. But as one's own "greatest hits" or portfolio of conditioned patterns and triggers become more familiar, the ID of them becomes less of a struggle. The experience becomes more often a matter of, "oh, that thing again," along with a perception of its degree of intensity and distractibility in the moment.

What is not required is some pristinely "empty" field in order to proceed to the main dropping-through practice. That's an idealistic notion, and an unrealistic one to boot; mind just inevitably generates stuff. With gradual skillfulness in knowing how one's own attention rolls, a sense develops of whether the weather in the field of mind is so stormy and distracting as to make the subsequent opening up an exercise in futility. So, decision-making as to how to proceed requires a little effort here. "Partly cloudy" is usually minimally acceptable weather in which to proceed to the next step in the sequence.

There are a dizzying variety of "vibe" practices from wisdom traditions across the globe and human history. I will ridiculously simplify that variety with but three different flavors, coming up: a "basic" attending, a "shiny keys" alternative, and the "where's the watcher" approach. There are those other multitudes of practices for you to investigate and perhaps dig into on your own. But my intention here is to focus on these for particular use as examples of attending to the prospect of emergent expansiveness, "fuzziness," and belonging. Yup, BFB.

Again, the approach is not the acquisition of anything, but opening to the possibility of an uncovering of some sense of big-M. In any of these practices, you may use the imaginal tactic of visualizing a release of the object of awareness—breath, a pattern set, whatever—into the broader field and then backing all the way back at "let it be and watch." It's like releasing that paper plane but focusing on the sky rather than the plane. What's that field like? What else is there?

Inevitably the plane comes to earth—ergo, you lose focus, awareness of the whole drops away to something else. Settle and rest a bit, then reset—back at the object (breath, set, thought) and...release, drop back to watcher/field—tend to the spaciousness. Be the space— notice how it feels in body, heart, mind, and especially the quality of awareness, of meta. Work in brief trials—a couple minutes tops, then rest in the breath, then back out.

It's inevitable that some specific, intrepid lookout for "big?" or a perception of loosened boundaries in time and self versus not or a wash of bliss may crank up. Our conceptual "BFB" prep work sets that up, and when some taste does emerge, the longing for a replay can intrude. Part of our "meta" skillfulness in these exercises involves managing that. A (intensely) watched pot won't boil, as everybody knows.

And of course, the dropping of effort at the "cooling down" denouement of practice is also included here. It requires the barest pivot and affords the goal of observing how the meditating mind shifts into "off the cushion" mode into the next moments of the day-to-day. Each of those ways of being with mind and Mind has its own kind of effort, pitfalls, and felt sense. As with prior routines, a bookending of noting the end of the sequence is helpful.

A New Twist on an Old Move: The Cosmic Air Filter

Before we move to the variations, let me introduce a tactic, akin to the "breathe into" and "drop into" skills, that can be of particular benefit in this big-M work. By now, the familiarity of the observed in-and-out breath can be used here to advantage. At a retreat a few years back, I snarkily once called it the "Cosmic Air Filter."[62]

While the tactic is employed in an imaginal way, its root is in quantum: the knowledge that absolutely everything is energy in its endless, multivariate forms. In the basic act of inhaling, we operate on that ocean of energy, pulling molecules of oxygen in, thereby nourishing our corpuscles and fueling us. With each breath we act on space and time, we bend the cosmos just a little; we twang the little strings of the vibratory whole. We breathe the big-M as we breathe ourselves.

So that simple act can generate a useful "cycling" routine in attending to the dance of separate self with cosmos—the little-m with the big-M. Breathing in can "contract" our attention to constructed self;

---

62   The retreat was in silence, otherwise, big laughs, I'm sure.

exhaling releases energy and attention out from constructed self to the all-encompassing Vibe felt as BFB.

The "cycling" tactic is most famously employed in the Buddhist compassion exercise known as "tonglen," itself a Tibetan mashup of two words ("gtong," meaning "send," and "len," meaning "take in")—"taking and sending," in the common translation. It's a practice of energy exchange—imagining "taking in" the suffering of another and then "sending out" goodness—compassion, kind wishes. As a physical parallel, the practice involves at its most basic the imaginal, visualized "inhaling" of the suffering of oneself or another—an act of wavicle empathy in its elemental form, really. Then, exhaling back out an energetic gift of sorts. We'll dive deeper into this in the next practice chapter. But I'm focusing here on that breathing tactic and a clever power in that in-out, that rhythm. Here's yet another, perhaps broadest utility of the simple act of breathing. With each in-breath, we gather up and contract awareness around the little-m, separate-self aspect of our parallel tracks of reality. With each out-breath, we expand awareness and open attention out to the big-M.

It's in to self, out to cosmos and its constituent wavicles. In to "me," out to "we."

Extra credit comes in getting that breathing routine humming, set in motion as its own cycling pattern, self/all, me/we, contracted matter to vibe connection. And then the tricky part: we step back from there, back to meta, and watch the cycling as we cycle. We can examine that state as we participate in it. We can watch for expansiveness, for a fuzzy opening out of the contracted self, for the warm hug of a sense of deeper connectedness. The attention will wander; an a-ha, then back to getting that breathing little-m/big-M cycle rolling again, and then back to meta.

As with any and all of the work we've pursued, keep in mind the duo of "watch-out-fors." One is that novel experiences are novel and can thus be provocative, even threatening in the "1.0 collapse" sense. The other is that the fruit of the practice at times may not be some glimpse of BFB, but what stuff routinely pops in to seemingly vandalize the exercise. That may be the more important stuff to tend to.

Vibe Practice I: Open Out, Go Meta

There's nothing fancy in this one; first we prepare awareness and our tuning in to the field of momentary mind, taking a gander at what stuff may be distracting and mugging for the camera. Phenomena and patterns may be present, but if the "weather system" is acceptable, we can move on to the main event—a simple opening to the whole field, including any and all stuff arising. This can be done with awareness in the basic "wide-angle" state, working in brief stretches (a couple of minutes at a time) of opening out the space of the field, as expanding as far as one can. This can seem befuddling; where does my awareness end? To this, I advise, don't get caught up in that narrative. It's the intentional act of directing awareness out without constraint that is key—casting an endless net out and stabilizing a sense of "big view" without too much itching to telephoto in on the stuff that comes and goes with that big view. With a little effort to "keep opened out" and some stability there, it's then time to go meta.

Our awareness directed to full landscape, we make the pivot to watching the watching. What is this state like? Is there a shift in the sense of spaciousness of the field of mind? Of a fuzzing of the boundary between regular "me-mind" and this state? Do I feel some different kind of connection? Or not much different or unique there for this particular moment?

In other words, any BFB going on? As I noted, the intention is to create some conditions in practice for witness, not to artificially manufacture or rationalize an experience of "bigness" or anything else. But this exercise can often open up that possibility: an "outside-in," felt sense of this expanded opening out of the full display is the goal.

Alternatively, we can plug in the "cycling" tactic described just above. We gather awareness "energy" in with each in-breath, then we open out with each out-breath, pushing energy and attention out beyond the self. It can be helpful to imagine awareness expanding sequentially out with each breath—like blowing a bubble of awareness. Then, the pivot to just watching and assessing that opened-out state, and note if and how something shifts in mind toward big-M.

We may practice in this way:

- 💬 Settle into a comfortable position; and prep: Here, We...Go (my intention, conditions permitting, is to open to bare awareness of the whole field and attend to its qualities);

- 💬 Engage a "warm-up plus," including a check of what pattern sets may be "active," and "meta" clarity of awareness; that being stable. Patterns and reactions may be present, but if not overly distracting, then proceed...

- 💬 Open out to fully to the "field"; consider walking out attention in steps to the space just around you, to the room, to the neighborhood, and ultimately out as far as your awareness can take you; allow some time to stabilize this.

- 💬 You may engage in this sequential opening out without regard to your breathing or can consider using the "cycling" breath tactic to "gather, then release" attention sequentially outward with each breath—observing rhythmic "snapshots" of the "local" effect on each in-breath, and that opened-out state as you exhale.

- Whether with bare observing, or using cycling, pull back to that "meta" mode: not just the field but the watching. Attend to the whole experience: the field, its stuff, and the felt sense of the watching itself. What's this like? What's the sense of size? Of boundary? Of connection?

- Work in a deliberate way in brief (few minutes, then rest) intervals. Open to the "full field" carefully with each interval, hopefully gaining some sense of holding that big view in a stable way; then let go back to meta and the effect in watching.

- As with every other exercise, be ready for the inevitable losses of attention that occur. Use your basic skills; without judgment, reset back on the breath, then proceed back as you see fit.

- Closing the practice here takes into account that opening out full to "meta" has actually been the central theme. So here, just move to letting go of any direction of awareness, just letting your mind be, resting back and observing mind settling back to its separate-self "steady state." There, we, are.

While any glimpse of aspects of BFB is possible and fortuitous, this exercise leans preferentially toward the "big," expansive aspect. One works in particular here with extending outward from the more "local" phenomena of body. The striving to open out farther than the usual "skin and in" quality of our daily experience by its nature works at attending to a bigger potential field to tune into. Using the "cycling" tactic helps draw attention to the capability of contracting and expanding our awareness in its rhythm.

Vibe Practice II: Shiny Keys

Hopefully that first variation created conditions for an outside-in view through the familiar tending to "stuff" and an opening to the Vibe all around. There's a New-Agey saying about these practices: they're like looking into a stream and peering through to the creek floor despite the distracting leaves floating by. For some, working with "leaves," be they individual entities or whole pattern sets, has become the favored practice. So, shifting to, "what else, besides the leaf," is not just novel but a struggle.

We can work on that. Building off our first variation, we'll introduce a critter in the field as a way of focusing awareness then pivot to "what else" as a way of distinguishing that space from the critter(s). This variation has always struck me as an inversion of the "shiny keys" technique parents may use with babies to draw their attention away. Here, we introduce the shiny keys, get locked in on them, then pull 'em away and let awareness open to the absence, to what else is there. It's clever, sometimes fruitful work.

While the "wait 'til something comes up" opening is certainly doable, for most folks, the pre-emptive selection of an object or pattern-set "key ring" generally is more effective, familiar target in that initial, concentrative aspect of this exercise. It can be as basic as the breath, or as multifaceted as a pattern set of a conflicted relationship with its layers of spin and backspin. But settle on something.

With that settled, we may practice in this way:

The usual prep and "warm-up" routine, then proceed to...

Open to a theme; best is one that feels familiar, immersing yourself in the full experience of the pattern set reaction. Breathe into it or "cycle" with it: in-breath to self, out-breath to the pattern set visualized as an entity in the field of mind. With some clarity perceived in the tuning into that pattern set...

- Imagine that set dissolving, or disappearing, or fading away in attention; open out to the sense of the field around the fading entity. Take the keys away and rest in observation of the whole. Imagine that entity fading, dissolving, being more transparent, then gone. You can use a basic, wide-angle observational mode, or...

- ...with the in-breath, contract awareness around the theme; with each out-breath, drop the theme and open out to "what else"—to the field, to the "not-the-theme." Gather energy in for attending to the keys, and then release the keys and open out to a broader awareness. Breathe "in" to shiny keys, out dissolving into Vibe.

- Take some time with this step—a couple minutes is reasonable—then, as before...

- Attend to the "meta" of observing the watching itself. What's this like? Where's the sense of boundary of "that stuff" versus "what else?" Observe for whatever does or doesn't arise—boundary shifts, expansiveness, unity.

- Work in that observation state until it degrades into distraction, or purposely rest back for a little bit. Then reintroduce the "theme," solidify attention on it, and then "pull the keys away" again, opening to the whole as before.

- Close the practice with the same "cool down" and TWA routines you are familiar with from the first variation.

This second variation, as it involves the abrupt shifting from a familiar wavicle aspect of little-m mind out to "everything else," can often work on that boundary-busting part of BFB. Moving from "it" (a part of "me") to "way out," operates in that fuzzy territory. I'm personally fond of this variation and work with it regularly as a go-to to open to Vibe. For me, the cycling of both breathing and its parallel in moving awareness often helps me in a felt sense of a softened, fuzzier hold on little-M, a relaxing of the day-to-day, separate Greg-ness.[63]

Vibe Practice III: Watcher, Meet Field

The last variation we'll try out is an old-school move, sometimes translated from the Tibetan into the mundane term, "looking," but a special and confounding kind: for proof of an observer separate from the field. There are many variations of these practices that are meant to generate by puzzlement a shift in experience, forcing the little-m mind out of its separate-self thinky state into the open space of big-M. A well-known flavor is the koan from the Zen branch of Buddhism. It's a question or idea that is intended to generate interior tension when approached logically, eventually "exhausting" self-generated analysis. In that petering out of any cortical answer, an opening to something present other than or beyond the cortex might just happen.

The "locate the watcher in the field of mind" trope, Waldo-like but with the treachery of no guy in stripes ever found, seems to me similar in use of observational futility to identify and thus separate watcher from field. In doing so, the exercise can thus reinforce a sense of union of watcher and field. I'm guessing this used to be a historically more effective "way in," but with copious written content on these practices being so ubiquitous in the West, there's a "spoiler alert" quality[64] that

---

63   It could just be the hyperventilating, but I don't think so.
64   "Where's Waldo? Psssst...you won't find him, he's everywhere! Or nowhere!"

could limit the utility of the practice. But it's actually worth working with if the exercise is worked on while taking that thought wavicle into account as a feeble distraction ("yes, I know what I'm supposed to (not) find...but let me look anyway and see what happens.")

I also have found a particular value: that this practice can complete the "trio" of variations in that it can operate preferentially to help open to a sense of belonging. While there's the risk of "oh, geez, there's no me I can find!" more likely the exercise tilts toward a warmer, "I'm an aspect of a bigger whole; I belong!"[65]

So, without undue peeking, we may practice in this way:

- 🍃 The usual prep and "warm up," yadda yadda yadda...

- 🍃 Open to the whole field. Observe in bare awareness or "cycle" with it: in-breath gathering to "local" self, out-breath out beyond to the field of mind. Breathe in "me," breathe out "we." Stabilize that sense of awareness. With some clarity sustained in that field-view...

- 🍃 Direct attention to the felt sense of awareness itself, with curiosity. Go "meta": watch for the watcher. Look for it, whether in a persistent way or with the cycling of each breath from "in" to "looking for" with each exhalation. As with the other exercises, work carefully and stabilize the sense of observing or cycling, then...

- 🍃 Pull back to attend to the effect of the whole experience. What's this like? What part of this field of awareness is "other," is "not home," barred from awareness? Or does it all "belong"? Keep returning to the looking, for a looker separate from the field, and then the effect it has on awareness.

---

65   But don't go looking for that either. Sheesh.

💬 The cooling down can proceed, dropping back to rest, and to put some gentle effort in observing mind settle back into its "little-m mode"...yet perhaps changed a bit in outlook. TWA.

Here are a couple of additional ideas and tips about this "looking" work. I'd suggest from my own trial and error that it helps to go eyes-closed for this one. An open visual field tends to overdrive a kind of outward sensory "searching" and a concrete, conceptual parking at, "the awareness is in my eyes," rather than a deliberate, patient examination of the mind-field. That attitude I hawked in the first discussion of basic sitting, of "beginner's mind," is especially good to start with here as a counterpoint to the conceptual stickiness lingering in 3.0 mind that, "I won't find the observer, so don't even bother."[66]

With that fresh curiosity of, "let's see what it's like this time?" an opening to BFB can arise, especially of a sense of unity and belonging. In the wonderment of where is some entity separate from the field doing the looking, there can arise a real-time taste of observer and field as one and the same. Rather than any alienating sense of "uh-oh, there's no 'me' there," a sense of "me may be an aspect of all," a true belonging to and part of Vibe, can emerge.

Well, That Sounds Easy...

The experiences that we just worked on setting the conditions for often require great persistence. Siddhartha Gautama's story, "he sat under a tree for forty-nine days until he got it," is the index case. Yet BFB can sometimes well up spontaneously—in a peak experience like witnessing a birth, or a nature scene, or even a fresh new view of a predictable or mundane moment. Sometimes it arises out of suffering. Eckhart Tolle, the author and lecturer who has written widely about

---

66 "Worst Easter egg hunt ever!"

his own meditative path, famously described an unbidden immersion into Vibe. He experienced a release from a contracted state of self in clinical depression, a relaxing of the sense of a "him" having that heaviness, and in its place an extended state of connected bliss that ultimately softened and stabilized but changed his outlook on being in the day-to-day world. BFB sort of just landed on him.

Other observers can get kind of overdramatic, even all hallelujah-chorus-preachy about this BFB thing, especially the "bliss" part. I worry that overdramatizing the subtle shift in awareness from a familiar, crystallized sense of self toward a "dissolving" of sorts actually hypes the state and diminishes it. "Self-defeating" would be a cute but ironic expression here, as this striving for bliss can actually be "self"-reinforcing. Weird is this whole thing, full of interesting ironies.[67]

It's a better plan to set some basic practice conditions for the experience to perchance happen, then practice with patience but without those outsized expectations of a peak moment. We live most all of life in the separate-self state, and that's where most of the suffering is, so mastering pattern sets, spins, and backspins are the paramount benefit of our work. Tasting the undercurrent Vibe will for most of us follow as we keep working on "cleaning the windshield." Moreover, becoming more aware of the undercurrent connection also softens the bumps of daily living. In that sense, both little-m and big-M are mutually reinforcing.

...But Not Always (Story Time!)

The bliss part sounds great, right? Not always, at least initially. The first taste of that dropping away of rigidly constructed self into some more transcendent state is a truly novel experience. Some react to a taste of one's own constructed self-sense loosening a bit not with

---

67   Yoda-esque, it is.

welcome, but instead 1.0 collapse fear—of a sterile emptying out or even a frightening annihilation. A volley into bliss doesn't necessarily get spun blissfully.

My first "immersion" experience snuck up on me, on a fine October evening as a "newbie" at a weekend meditation retreat in Northern California. I'd had a rough day on the inner prairie[68] with reactivity and patterning cluttering up things. The struggle pushed me to work-work-work on the "material" getting in the way of aspired-to clear attention on my grand staircase up to samadhi—a rookie tactic.

Walking off my frustration in the chilly evening, I barely noticed the waning light of sunset over rolling hills—not necessarily sublime, but just right for there and then. An out-of-left-field notion occurred to pause my cognitive cement-mixing and just attend to the beauty of the scene. I let go of my mental gymnastics and rested in the simplicity of watching the sun go down from a pedestrian bridge on the walking path.

What felt like a warm hole opened up right between my eyes. The sensation was subtle at first, then opening out broadly, and truly novel. Patterns in mind sort of floated with my usual tight clutch of them instead relaxing, and spreading out, then...harder to express. "They melted into everything else" approaches it. Mind felt not emptied nor destroyed but immersed in a state of wholeness with what I'd perceived as "not-me." Tightness, rules, constructions were not overcome as much as subsumed by a "knowing" in the head, radiating out, and an associated felt state of warmth in the heart of deep belonging, wholeness, affiliation.

Yet it also felt incredibly unfamiliar in terms of my grooved-in perceptions of myself, my mind, Me with a capital M. Where'd it go? Where'd I go? The experience stayed and hummed awhile; I had enough sense to let it. It faded with the setting sun.

---

68   My mind-field was a mine field.

I went back to my room, vaguely shocked by the occurrence. I wrote it off, minimized it, tried to rest a little before the evening teaching session, in which "breaking silence" is allowed in otherwise quiet retreat conditions. My fervent hope was for some generic chatter on breathing, monkey-mind, whatever, followed by a quit exit back to my room to close out this weird evening.

No luck. The issue of opening to the "empty" state somehow became the hot topic. As some of the more seasoned participants recounted their own tastes of that openness, hearing these testimonies opened me up, but in a fragile way. The "what happens to me?" volley kicked up and felt overwhelming. It was certainly not blissful: I was cooking on my own dread of dissolution, of either/or: my familiar, separate lump o' Greg versus a drowning in the cosmic soup. I can now interpret after the fact that a new sense of "home" was emerging for me. But at the time, a feared collapse to 1.0 was occurring in response to a hairy new serve in my court.

My heart started to hurt—like a panic attack, but fight more than flight. Some 3.0 chatter charged in, pumping a kind of web of rash judgments, unusual stuff for this typically accepting, reasonable wavicle: these people are deluded; I'm a fool. This is bullshit. Shame on all of it. I felt a magnetic pull to escape. Not wanting to look foolish, I tuned out a little emotionally, got through it, then scuttled back to my cubbyhole dorm room, heart rate remaining up and mind on fire.

The rest of the evening was an interesting, now memorable one. I couldn't sleep, so I meditated in a very simple way, not striving to recreate nor to disprove the sunset splash into the oceanic. Wavicles of body, heart, and head ebbed and flowed. The "opportunity" afforded by this cascade put me right in the spot I needed to be in observing those as phenomena, with an open awareness of the host of defensive "moles" that were popping up and a simple sense that I should just watch and not whack them. An aspect of the blissful somatic/emotional state did also sneak back in—enough to be apprehended, but in a quieter, familiar kind of comfort and peacefulness. I knew enough not to chase that any more than I should whack away at the negative and fearsome phenomena. I was letting the road to settling play out and starting to taste some acceptance of this new outlook.

For all my magical fear of "self dissolving," what occurred instead was a travelogue of the various constructions of me, some especially radioactive in the midst of their being observed. They, and I, didn't disappear. Most of all, the sense of alienation I dreaded, perhaps even concocted, was what had dissolved. It was replaced with a profound sense that this "peace," this belonging sensation, was a birthright. I was mindful, but just hadn't been aware of it.

And then some peaceful sleep came, albeit at three o'clock. An interesting night, indeed. (And no "Mary Had A Little Lamb" within earshot.)

My separate-self construction survived and lives to this day, but was/ is attended to in a different, less bound-up way, at least part of the time. There was a kind of animation to my experience that has since ebbed and flowed. The qualities of spaciousness, of a softening of the rigid boundaries of "my mind," and of a felt belonging, are routinely re-lost and regained in my unfolding experience, as for most anyone who works this thing. That's the imperfect reality of our minds down in the weeds: the contracting around our self-construction is a recurrent inevitability, each ebb and flow of experience and its pathway for us to hold lightly and observe.

Each bump affords an opportunity for little-m and big-M. For me, "what else is there?" was a fruitful drop-into practice. Mine is not a particularly special example. Go and have yours. Each identification of a pattern set, or series of them, allows not just for observation of the wavicle but also for what that wavicle is swimming in. Try to rest in that space, immersed and observant.

CHAPTER 15

Home Again, Home Again: Some Final Words on Mindfulness

We made it! We've chugged through a practical but comprehensive sequence of concepts and practices to go about the complex act of examining, understanding, and living a life in deeper awareness.

We started with Part I's practices in holding, losing, and regaining awareness in a basic way via the breath. We then worked methodically in Part II through the stuff in the field—physical, emotional, conceptual, and the faculty of the watching itself. Exercises involving our individual experience immersed in the big "field" filled out Part III.

The practices are meant to be cumulative with each additional practice adding a little more to work with. Meditation is most often used in a scheduled way, but can also be moment-, event-, or challenge-specific, as in developing a preparatory sitting routine for work or a go-to routine in moments of craving or anxiety. Many practitioners find meditation practice as an incremental collector's walk, picking up a tool kit of skills and insights along the long way, saving and cherishing those that serve each of us best according to our singular temperaments and needs.

Yet all of that complexity may seem unwieldy or overwhelming for some. Examining the way mind works from a decidedly different framework, or any framework at all, is not for everybody.[69] So, here's a final swing at the question...why should we examine experience?

Yeah, Why Do That?

There has been a developing emphasis in the current media on understanding the primacy of our early experience in shaping our later minds. This is a good thing.[70] Yet the opportunity awaits for adults not just to look back, but to grow forward cognitively and psychologically. In a deliberate way, we can and should cultivate the ability to grow in wisdom all though life, especially through adulthood.

Biologically, we're built with the capabilities of apprehension and comprehension. Memory, intelligence, and the obscure but essential process of gaining wisdom through conscious contemplation and unconscious processing all are privileged attributes worthy of appreciation.

Through the sharpening of our skills in awareness training, we can become familiar with the core details of our inner "home." We can work carefully in more advanced practices to understand the activities in that home in pattern and process, to master familiarity of aspects of our moment-to-moment sequence of events. Knowing the patterns of impact, reaction and counteraction, and better managing our reactions, we navigate the "matter" world with more skill.

Our "separate-self" patterning and sequencing having become demystified and more transparent, it ceases to operate out of

---

69   Actually, I take that back—it should be, but many don't know it.
70   If only focusing more societal resources on early life would be the result. Our public investments are currently more skewed to selfishly preserving security and comfort for aging Boomers. Ok, indeed.

awareness and softens, if not fades. Those obstructions of separate self more out in the open, awareness gains the opportunity to open beyond the contracted self to deeper connections and belonging, if that is of interest and inquiry.

Any practice, however simple or rococo, can be fruitful if practiced with effort and intention. The humble breathing awareness practice, an elemental stress management tool, is itself complete and very potent. Beyond the calming features of watching the breath and attending to the body and heart, we encounter the inevitability of losing and regaining attention and the eventual learning of what pulls attention away, drowns it in narrative, or otherwise jams us up. As with the core tactic in regaining lost attention, there need not be any judgment. Find and use what works best.

My own meditative "career" has warbled over time. I've run extended periods of more complex observation tactics, especially when I've become aware of some troublesome current inner dynamic or outer conflict that signals me to dive in a bit more deeply. Those periods have been intermixed with stretches of the simple purity of walking my focus out to the breath and working with that to great benefit. Sometimes there are "deep" days and "keep it simple" days, depending on the time and energy available to me. Each individual eventually gains a personal feel for what works in the whole and in the moment.

The core expectation is of enhanced capacity of awareness, of what is occurring in the real time of each of our moment-to-moment lives. It prepares for and reduces the tension of our uncertainty. It makes us less likely to cling to stuff past its due-date, run from stuff that we have trouble holding, or ignore stuff we should pay attention to. In short, training our attention supercharges our adaptive capability, a potential attribute just waiting there to be optimized.

And, simply, most people just report feeling and doing better from day to day when they meditate. There's that.

A "child's eye" of a fresh awareness does not preclude attending with our "separate-self" faculties to the "matter" aspects of being in the world, to the day to day navigating of wants, needs, complex relationships, lost keys, and floods.[71] We could use a little more individual contemplation in the world. And a lot more belonging.

So, that's why.

Can I Stop Now? Sure, But...

We've covered the basic ground of basic awareness meditation fairly thoroughly. We've got maps to use. We've worked through a series of sequenced practices, starting with the basics and building on those skills out to a fuller view of the entities that operate in the moment-to-moment mind. This a common stopping point for books and workbooks on stress management-based meditation practice. For many readers, this may be the pith of what you're looking for.

In that spirit, take it and run if this is sufficient for your goals or needs. It's just fine to park here. Review the practices, stick with each one for a little while to get the hang of it, and construct your own routine or routines for everyday use. And practice, practice, practice. Be patient, curious, and humble about the variety of experiences that occur in your "home" from day to day. Look for the benefit off the cushion.

Yet we can go deeper. The identification of states of experience that we've worked on to date implies that experiences and patterns are static, pinned down. We've gotten very good at witnessing one drawing of that stick-figure guy in the kineograph "flip book," but not so much the experience of movement when we flick through the pages. The vignette above, the flip book, and your own experience

---

71   The old joke about the grumpy, drowned dude at the pearly gates—"but I sent you a boat!"—is informative here.

so far, I'll bet, show that experience is always in motion. Events, reactions, and judgments come and go, and morph with time and additional input.

Practical Mindfulness mostly addresses the basic construction of our minds with a little taste of the deeper reality to start attending to. For some of us, diligent practice allows for a gradual unearthing and demystifying of the distracting, conditioned stuff that obscures a deeper dive into Vibe.

For many others, that wavicle safari can be more complicated. The phenomena of body, heart, mind, and awareness don't always (or perhaps ever) just explode into the field. You may have noticed that combinations of each of those categories from our initial mapping of mind stuff often run in predictable, repeating patterns. Using the OS map, we can observe certain emotional 2.0 stuff mostly always kick up partners in OS 3.0 storytelling, and occasionally even 1.0 threat. Example: summer party, maybe too much beer among the assembled: you get pushed in the pool along a few others...you feel cold, you get ticked at the fool that did the deed; you remember a fleeting moment of fear of drowning the first time we got shoved in as a kid. There's a pattern for you.

As we examine the wavicles, then the combos and patterns of them more closely, we actually can encounter more complexity: our patterns of experience often generate a reaction—a "spin" on the pattern. Back poolside: humiliated and rageful at your wet clothes, dead cellphone, and the giggles and guffaws of the throng throwing each other overboard, you lose your cool and unleash a string of expletives and threats. Your tirade: there's another pattern, a "spin."

And we maybe even find a reaction to that reaction—a "backspin." One last lap: your blowup garners a mix of responses, from "chill out!" to concern for your well-being to condescending "poor baby" commentary. It's not the first time you've gone Vesuvius over a surprise moment of bad press; a feeling of shame kicks in, a wishful desire to disappear. A flash memory of a big brother picking on you whizzes by, as does breaking some Legos afterward. There's some heavy backspin.

Moments occurs with their individual imprints, reactions, and secondary reactions. Minds are complicated that way, but this is where applying our observational capacities can suss out the patterns and sequences. Yes, these things often operate in steps, sequences that can identified and even anticipated. The better we know our patterning, not just the wavicles roaming our individual fields but their habits and running mates, the less rattled we are when they inevitably show up. And the more likely we can drop though them to deep states of calm and belonging.

Final Thought I: One Last Clip (Of a Long Movie)

As I'm finishing up, let me pivot back to the personal for a couple of riffs. A novel approach to this, "we're immersed but we're also observing" thing occurred to me in watching my own reactivity recently.

I'll set the scene: driving to work, I was toodling along with my lovely view of the springtime Sierra foothills mugging for my attention. Shoots of young grass were vibrant green on the hillside, soon to go golden with the California summertime. The hiking trail snaking up the hill to my right was so familiar that I could place myself anywhere along it and be there in mind. Big ol' oak trees anchoring the hillside were like old stalwarts in that tilted park, their early leaves gently fluttering, even dancing if I imagined it.[72]

---

72   Yes, this may seem familiar. Turn back to the beginning of Chapter 1 if you wish.

A quick imprint occurred. Even a bit of a "dropping into" glimpse into deeper awareness, as is an occasional thing on my commute. But there was also some taking for granted of my fortunate surroundings and a quick contracting back to "little-m" mind of a shrink on a mission.[73]

Approaching a stop sign, I pulled up behind a large, late-model SUV—an Exploitation, or an Emasculade, or something like that—and expected the driver to tap the brakes, slow up briefly, and then head on through the otherwise empty intersection. But he was not playing along. Through his heavily tinted glass I could make out an angrily self-involved dude barking into his cellphone and gesticulating wildly. I was trapped behind him full stop, queued up at this stop sign, busy me an unwilling participant in this new mind moment.

I checked my immediate, irritable reaction to his self-centered act encroaching on my smooth passage to the office. His me-first behavior generated, ironically, a reciprocal contracting of my own mind around (my) self. What's with this $^#*@ guy? How dare he? I got stuff to do! In grievance, I simmered a little and tried to observe the simmering.[74]

Resonating with the prior scene, I pondered the moment and a bigger-picture issue emerged. Yes, I went a little meta...watching my reaction, I contemplated how we can reinforce the contraction around the painful moment and let any embeddedness in a broader Vibe easily drop away to our self-only perception. Whatever this blasted connection to Vibe is, it's really easy to lose the signal.

As I prepared to gun around him with possible use of my middle finger as a turn signal, I looked up at the surrounding hills still visible

---

73 If four tardy chart notes and twenty minutes on hold with an insurance company can be grandly called a "mission."

74 Amazing how writing a book on this stuff reminds you to be more attentive yourself!

at the intersection. An idea popped in. What would this little scene look like from up there on the hill?

An alternative to an "it's my life" view in the driver's seat can be approached from that observer's hillside view, starting the scene at your birth and ending it with your demise. Imagine witnessing the time course of a life, not from inside your skull, but instead from up on that hill. You can watch it like a trip that runs over time or one of those time-lapse movies of a mountain as the weather changes over the seasons. From that view, the "me" is actually not a persistent "thing," but an "era"—the era in which the quarks and bosons are organized into the complex entity called Greg, or Kelly, or Rajiv, or Shauntae, or you.

But for a (maybe chilling, at first) moment, recognize that the movie is but a clip in a much longer film, not just a contained little piece with its own theme song and rolling credits.[75] Sitting from that hill, picture an introductory, cinematic sweep—a pretty long one, really—in which those quarks and bosons have yet to organize into the self-aware protoplasm called you. There's a long shot of landscape without you,[76] a tender, green you-shoot sprouts out of the ground, solidifying to a blade of grass, a beautiful flower, or a mighty oak, or maybe something less iconic or more fragile; and then fading off, inevitably over time, going to ground, fertilizer for the next eras, the next clips in the long-running show. After your scene, another endless stretch of movie featuring other eras with their own expositions, plot twists, climaxes of various sorts, denouements, and curtains closing. Like you, their quarks go to ground, too—still in the scene, but not organized forward and more self-aware.

From this view, we are embedded in the bigger cinema. Telephoto of "my life" becomes the landscape view of "my era in big-M Mind" or perhaps a personal scene in an endless film running.

---

75 The "gaffer" can be your Uncle Louie.
76 Get more popcorn.

Hit "play." The Shauntae era, the you era, the me era, each lasts a while. We can see changes in physical shape driven by the march of time. Behold your cute-cartoonish, big-cranium'ed toddlerhood; your ripe adolescence; the fullness and strength of your peak of young adulthood; the middle-age changes in shape, volume, and tone; the inevitable withering in your old age, should you get there. Then, a quiet demise: a bag of bones.

Less apparent is the inner script during that era, your era. Imagine, like that time-lapse footage, the possible flowering of cooing to early childhood reactivity, to the concentration of you the fourth grader on math homework; to a developing self of you-in-the-world as you hit twelve, then twenty and onward. The era of yourself could and should be just getting revved-up at twenty. Self-awareness and wisdom in understanding of one's immersed place in the cosmos can and should morph and shift and deepen through the era of your conscious life.

That's your home. Take good care of it.

Final Thought II: About Finality

A phrase caught my eye recently in a paper on neuroplasticity, the term for the brain's propensity to change and reallocate functions and processes in response to life events as we go along. It's a relatively novel area of investigation; even just thirty years ago, we docs in training were taught that the brain is pretty much set like concrete by late adolescence. We now know differently.

The interesting snippet from the paper: that mental events are *"temporary coalitions of synapses that form and disperse."*

It's an unusual perspective, but nods to the inevitability of patterns of matter and mind coming, then going. The ocean of Vibe is awash with bumps. And with each bump happening, our little-m selves form and, yes, disperse.

With self-awareness, we gain an understanding of an ever-changing home in this way and even make new wavicles for it. As a final aside, this may be the only, tangential way I can buy into the "reincarnation" idea. To be honest, I've tended to judge that idea harshly as it sounds like a human yearning to defend against the most profound grieving of all—of one's own end. It seems to me an aspirational stretch, my "special packet of soul," airmailed to some next bodily destination.

In the Latin breakdown, the term "reincarnate" can be framed as "make into a form, again." Maybe I'm just trying to make it work, but I can ally with that, a little. Not as a "special packet of soul," but a simpler co-metabolism of constructed self and the undercurrent Vibe in which it lovingly belongs. It perhaps stays unified, but perhaps it dissolves and reforms. That separate self can make a difference in its era, and hopefully a beneficial effect, one that outlives the humble but remarkable era of sentient you, of self-aware me.

Maybe "pro-incarnation" works better as a term. Each bump generates more new reality, new little-m construction out of the big-M soup of Vibe. Each little snippet of film in our separate-self eras represents the sausage-making of new wavicle production, of incarnation. It's a blessing as well as a job, and even a responsibility. Being alive and awake can hurt, but it's a rare state, and not one to waste.

Ultimately, as we know better the complex aspects of our moment-to-moment sequence of events, the patterns of impact, reaction, and counteraction, we navigate the matter world with more skill live in and contribute to the deeper Vibe, the broadest home in which we belong.

Everything, every single thing, becomes...home.

Practically Finished

Let me express my gratitude for your effort and attention to reading and using *Practical Mindfulness*. I hope it becomes your go-to guide and resource for a lifelong routine in practicing meditation to improve your life. At the very least, hopefully it's offered a novel spot from which you may consider the workings of your individual experience.

In the no-nonsense, practical spirit of the book, let's crowdsource this project of bringing more mindfulness to more of us.

Please consider visiting www.practicalmindfulness.com, which offers access to my various social media exploits.

- Consider tuning into the "Practically Mindful Moment" podcast, dropping in late 2020. I'll be briefly summarizing some practical tips, tactics and troubleshooting on all things mindful. The podcasts are bite-sized—from two to ten minutes—to give you a quick something to ponder, add to your knowledge base on mindfulness, or wow your friends with at parties.

- Feedback is welcome: post a review on Amazon or Goodreads; drop me an email (drsaz@surewest.net).

- At the website, I hope you'll peruse my posts on the *Practical Mindfulness* Blog, where I elaborate briefly on mindfulness and its application in our current times.

There's one further application of mindfulness to engage some readers in. You don't have to be an expert to share the basics of meditation to share the goodness. If you get the sense that the information and practices laid out in this book are not only of benefit to you but are worth sharing in your own role as a health professional, teacher, caretaker, or parent, well, that's a good idea.

An Appendix You May Want to Keep After All

I've spent some time and effort distilling the basic "starter pack" for teaching breath meditation, "teaching the teachers" both in terms of elementary school staff and medical residents. Please consider reviewing and using the Appendix which follows this afterword. It offers some helpful information for those professionals and caretakers that not only want to use mindfulness themselves but also provide some basic training in breath meditation and the "breather" tactic to their own patients, students, and loved ones. It walks through the how to's of addressing questions about the practice, a sample script based on my own work in with medical trainees in providing this teaching to their patients. You'll also find some handouts that you can use in clinics and classrooms.

Thanks for reading and participating.
GCS

See Om, Do Om, Teach Om: Spreading the Goodness

Mindfulness is breaking out everywhere lately. Once thought a fringe-y practice, meditation has recently found its way into healthcare organizations, schools, the corporate workplace, prisons, and spiritual settings. If not yet quite a cornerstone of stress management, it's a welcome and growing application in many arenas of modern, often stressful public life.

We got some numbers. The CDC reports that the overall percentage of American adults who have tried meditation has increased (in 2019) to around one in seven (14 percent), about threefold more than in 2012 (4.5 percent). That's terrific, until you consider that the other 86 percent of Americans don't meditate.

Other statistics to compare that to: 94 percent of Americans know how to ride a bike. About 72 percent know how to cook decently. 25 percent can play at least a little bit of piano. It's admittedly much higher than those who can tango (max 1 percent or less), but lower than those who can juggle (21 percent). My educated guess is that meditators actually make better jugglers. I'm not sure about the tango.

It's also finally breaking through some old stereotypes in terms of what entrepreneurial types call "barriers to entry." These include mistrust in the validity of a subjective, hard-to-assess interior experience. Another is an uncomfortable association with religiosity: meditation as an esoteric, mystical, even cultish activity. There are some gnarly old xenophobic roots there about Eastern practices and a resultant, unfounded sense of threat to some in established Western religious traditions.

Despite all that, meditation is being increasingly being adopted as a helpful adjunct to traditional spiritual practices. According to the helpful survey folks at Pew Research, 40 percent or more of Americans who identify as belonging to an organized religion now include a meditative component in their prayerful activities.

The positive health implications are also increasingly clear. The evidence for mindfulness practices helping manage anxiety, pain, and insomnia is strong. There's good data for reductions in hypertension, coronary artery disease, and symptoms of PMS in meditators. Cognitively, there is measurable improvement in memory and reduced distractibility in learning. Teachers are becoming much more tuned in at this point, with terrific programs for teacher training in mindfulness and apps that target basic meditation in age-appropriate ways.

Nevertheless, many in some "people" professions—ok, let's take my profession—have been a little slow to catch on. Less than 5 percent of physicians recommend meditation to their patients, let alone teach them some basic form of the training. I get it; we're busy and increasingly overwhelmed by the current burdens of medical practice. There's the practical obstacle of squeezing even basic meditation skills training into many docs' already over-subscribed treatment visits. The blizzard of documentation expectations in modern medicine amplifies the storm.

But regardless of the possible reasons for stiff-arming it, meditation training makes our jobs easier. Patients become more collaborative with us in their care. Stress-related impacts on a vast variety of medical and psychological conditions improve. It's a valuable tool to incorporate into education in medical and other interpersonal settings—starting with our personal self-care routines.

My intention, then, in this practical chapter in a practical book is to practically put myself out of business, mindfulness-training-wise. Yes, you too can teach others the basics of beginning meditation. And for the reasons above, you probably should.

Who, Me? (You Too Can Goo-Roo)

There's an old expression in medical training: "see one, do one, teach one." It nods to the expectations for an unrealistically rapid development of competence expected of physician trainees and their mentors in all sorts of interventions in the hospital environment. Draw blood? See one, do one, teach one. Find and successfully hit a wrist artery for a blood gas sample at four in the morning? S1-D1-T1. Inebriated, combative patient in the ER needs a spinal tap? Un-huh. (I nailed that one, but on the third stick, after seeing a few done. Sorry, dude.)

As an aside, the best chance of not winding up as a guinea pig for an inexperienced trainee in a training hospital is actually calendar-based: don't get sick in July. Medical training residencies traditionally start, you guessed it, on July 1. There's a lesson for you.

Assuming you've read the book up to this point and engaged diligently in the practices I've described, you've got a bit of "see one" and "do one" under your belt already. Congratulations! "Teach one" is not a stretch, and it may well be an additional skill set that will help you as a parent, teacher, doctor, nurse, therapist, or workplace trainer. Even outside those obvious professions, most all of us have played "teach," starting informally as kids on the playground, through study groups in school, and into roles as parents and mentors. We teach our kids which fork to use when, proper free throw technique, and manners when the grandparents visit.

Conveying the basics of beginning meditation for stress management does not require an advanced degree. By all means, recommend the book too; but keeping it simple, you can do this.

A Basic Definition, an Attitude Check, Then an Offer

Whether in a medical consultation room, a psychotherapy office, a classroom, or a conference room, proposing an activity that invites examination of one's own mind is often a very personal "ask." It can be an intrusive and risky-sounding invitation for some. So a brief explanation of what meditation is (and is not) is an important prerequisite to any offer to teach or refer.

You've heard me make the basic stress management case already—to you. I'd try to keep it more basic and unadorned when discussing it in person:

> *Meditation is a way to get better at focusing on what's happening in the moment. That includes our inner experience, as well as what's occurring outside and around us.*

> *When we work on that basic kind of observation, with practice we gradually get better at managing difficult feelings and experiences that come up—like anxiety, pain, and sadness. We can gain more control over all of that, which is a good thing.*

Before I engage in any possible "contracting" about learning to meditate, I feel strongly that the "attitude check" for the work is essential to set from the get-go. It's actually a strongly persuasive factor in how prospective meditators decide.

There's one really important aspect of meditation: an attitude thing. It goes best with an attitude of curiosity about how our minds work. Not so much with an attitude of having to "get it right" or judgment about how it's going.

In fact, it's important to have some humility and even compassion for ourselves when it gets difficult, because that'll absolutely happen sometimes. So we try to drop off the judgy attitude to start. And just watch it if or when it comes up—it's just another thought to distract us, right?

Sometimes the response to this plea for keeping an open mind about opening the mind is met with a thousand-mile stare, especially among strivers who want meditation to be another game to win. It's hard for many of us to shake the competitive conditioning we've grown up with, from sports to grades to promotions. But there can are be a kind of relief, a permission to let go of the driving and the striving, and just tune in. I think the "walk in the landscape" metaphor helps reinforce this practice as play, as exploration, with a side of calm and relief. Usually, there's buy-in to make an effort at this nonjudgment aspect of the practice. Then, we ask (not demand, or shame into):

So...sound like something you'd like to try? Got any questions?

Usually, there are questions. Not surprisingly, some misconceptions too. So, anticipate. Here are some golden oldies.

- Most people start by watching their breathing as practice. You can count the breaths if you like or just observe the air going in and out.

- It's absolutely normal to lose track, sooner or later. It happens to everybody, and it's nothing to beat yourself up about. We just notice we've lost track, then go back to watching.

- Meditation's completely different from "thinking." It's actually about watching. Watching what happens to some part of our experience, or even all of it.

- It's not about stopping our minds from having thoughts. No one can really do that. We can work to reduce how much we add to the story with more distracting thoughts. But having thoughts is not "doing it wrong." That's just how minds are.

- Usually you can start with a couple minutes, and then go a little longer as you get the hang of the basic watch it/lose it/"oh"/back to watching it thing. It'll take some time and practice, but most people really benefit over time when they stick with it. Consider, say, four weeks of effort.

Then, no pressure selling. This isn't a kitchen appliance or a timeshare. I also offer information on some commonly used, helpful guided meditation apps out there. If there's agreement, we schedule some teaching time. Or if there's a little time in the current visit (I'd say ten minutes as a minimum), I launch into some brief teaching.

The briefest instruction for a short, shared, guided practice, right there and then, can be helpful to lower the bar:

We can try it right now, if that's ok.
We'll go for a minute or so. I'll meditate with you.
Get comfortable but alert, like this.

(Sit up straight with both feet on the floor and hands on your knees, to model a reasonable position to follow.)

Pick a spot on the floor to train your eyes on, or close them if you want.
Select a place to watch your breath—nose, throat, or belly. Watch yourself breathing in, then breathing out.
At some point, you will lose track of that. When you do, without fuss, go back to watching the in and out of breathing.

I'll let you know when we're halfway done. Ok, let's start.

I've been accused of using something called my "Mister Rogers voice"—a badge of honor!—in indicating the halfway mark, as well as some accentuated wheezing as a modeling sound for deep breaths. I often add a quietly intoned...

"when you lose track, it's ok—just go back to watching your breath."

Then, call time. Then, to a quick check-in...

"So, what was that like? Notice anything? Feel any different?"

...which not only reinforces your interest in the individual's experience, but also models an aspiration for that individual to notice, too. A little "meta" mentoring, right there out of the gate.

I usually offer patients a handout (also available at practicallymindful. com) that has directions for basic breath meditation on one side and that lovely puzzle graphic on the other.

If I have more time to spare, or in that scheduled training, I use that puzzle graphic to walk through a quick overview of the five basic components of our awareness that should be familiar to you by now:

- Physical stuff... (inside sensations, of which the breath is the first and best target, and outward sense experiences)

- Emotional stuff (with kids, it helps to identify it as "weather inside"—adults, too)

- Thought stuff...this can be a novel idea to some, that thoughts are "stuff I notice," rather than personalized, fully owned aspects of self. They come and go

- The "field" in which that other stuff is coming and going; subtler to observe; useful to frame as "open? Contracted and tight? Spacious or full of the other stuff?"

💬 The "watcher"..."that's you, the observer, the one part
that really stays put, something you can get to know and
return to"

This way to visualize awareness as a kind of field or landscape
organizes things a bit. From that broader picture, I identify the
breath as but one physical thing in the landscape to pick as a target
of observation, and a really good one, verified by millennia of folks
trying stuff out. It is common to some experience some calming just
through the witness of the breath, without any specific directive to
slow it down or deepen it.

It's the same with an alternative target:

"Pull your attention out to how your whole body feels."

We tend toward relaxation of muscle tension once we acknowledge it.

Whether it's a quick run through or a longer tutorial, I try to spend
a final moment or two on next steps and expectation. If your patient,
student, or peer is interested, suggest a commitment of daily practice
for a stretch of time. Kick around ideas about a favored or protected
place and time for practice. I often suggest that a reminder alarm on
the smartphone or laptop can be a good reinforcer. It's also a good
idea to mutually "contract" to follow up at a subsequent meeting, or
via a scheduled phone or text contact in a couple of weeks.

A Couple More Options to Teach (Recycling Is Good)

The basic breath-watching meditation routine is plenty effective as
a tool to teach in clinical offices, classrooms, and the other settings
I've mentioned. Beyond that, I've encouraged my family medicine
trainees to branch out a little based in their own interest level and in
response to particular patient needs. You can, too!

Some incorporate the "trey" or "three-pointer" variation with their patient teaching. You remember that one, right? It was simple structuring of the breath observation—breath arcing up, out-breath arcing back down, and adding right there a quick observational snapshot of the full physical self, then to the next in-breath. This scheduled "feel your body" direction can help folks who struggle to tune into physical states of experience and suffering unless/until the states are severe. Earlier awareness of building pain or discomfort can allow them to respond earlier as needed with their own treatment or seeking it out, and in many cases of chronic, waxing/waning states (fatigue, chronic pain, headache, muscle tension) can cultivate some adaptation and tolerance of these moments with a more insightful sense of one's own "threshold" for action, rather than a binary "ignore it or head to the ER" model.

One other routine that I will recycle here for professionals to teach to others is that "Mindful Breather" routine just inflicted on you a mere chapter back. I'll include a handy handout on this one below as well as at the website. As it's a step beyond that first teaching of breath meditation; it requires a little overview of that puzzle graphic (or at least a quick lesson on our physical, emotional, and thinky components of self and observing with the mind's eye).

I've found that patients dig the "Breather" as a superior form of the stereotypical but functional, "just count to ten" direction when in states of explosive irritability, anxiety, or pain. It works to tend to the emergent wavicle of the moment in a systematic, four-breath (minimum) checklist, which allows for some fuller understanding of the effect (body, heart, head, watcher). In doing so, it imposes a brief interlude, perhaps a little longer than counting to ten, that hits a pause button on the novelty of the experience. The angry text or email is less likely to be sent; a screaming jag at one's naughty kid or wayward life partner may be reconsidered just by having been taught to take a mindful breather.

And this virtuous cycle can spread. For example, parents who gain facility with this tactic may teach their own children. Like a benevolent virus, this mindfulness is.

Teachers who have introduced basic breath meditation to their students can advance the "mindful breather" training. Many school districts finding legal and educational dead-ends in seclusion/ suspension/expulsion policies for students losing control in classrooms have been setting up alternative cool-down "recovery rooms," staffed with teachers and/or aides. Basic breath meditation skills are routinely used; the "breather" is another, more targeted way to help revved-up kids pull it back together and return to their classroom without punishment or shaming.

Bring Along the Family! (Or Class, Or Group)

While I've directed most all of the content and exercises in *Practical Mindfulness* as individual endeavors, buddying up for practice can be a powerful reinforcement, as with exercise. Friends or couples can have a shared sitting. The basic breath work directions are actually accessible to kids as young as four or five. A sequential mindfulness curriculum that I developed for elementary school kids, 123 Focus, is a little more structured, walking participants (teachers/parents) and kids through breath meditation out to fuller observation of the landscape. I've made that open source, also at the website, for the whole clan to partake in. Families that wheeze together, um, are pleased together. Or something.

A Warning Label

Who should not come along for the lesson? The basic stress management-based breath meditation that I've suggested for your use and conveying to others is most always well received and helpful. Yet there is a nominal but real risk for some individuals, a risk to monitor for and get some expert consultation about.

For folks who are in midst of or have recently been struggling with severe psychiatric illness, it's best to have their mental health specialist (psychiatrist, psychologist, and/or therapist) weigh in on the appropriateness of starting a meditation practice. That includes those with deeper clinical depressive syndromes, with disordered thought content and/or process (psychosis), and with recurring dissociative states (often a feature of Post-Traumatic Stress Disorder).

Lastly, basic meditation can actually be of help in managing the frustrations that arise for individuals in the early stage of dementia. But as dementia progresses, attention itself can become impaired, making mindfulness training itself another frustrating exercise.

Diving into deeper meditative work, beyond the practices I've laid out in *Practical Mindfulness*, can risk springing a painful opening to intense personal patterning and even traumatic re-experiencing for some individuals. That's a separate issue and book, and it's important to note that getting guidance with that meditative work is a reasonable option.

Nevertheless, there are those with traumas, often suffered early in life, that got buried psychologically: "repressed" is the term for those memories that on rare occasion can erupt unbidden into current awareness. Events in the current day can sometimes trigger the whole past mess into the moment. Even basic mindfulness training, as it does invite an examination of one's experience, can very occasionally trip that wire. The follow-up contact I recommended to check on compliance with and the results of the initial training should also include a check-in on any difficulties that arise with the practice.

We Sorta Glossed Over "Do One"

In guiding patients through even the basics of a practice about an interior, subjective state, nothing can replace your direct engagement in basic meditation. In imparting this bit of advice, I am reminded of the classic advice of the esteemed educational consultant, one Marjorie Jacqueline Bouvier Simpson:

> *Marge: I could teach piano classes or something.*
>
> *Lisa: But you don't play the piano.*
>
> *Marge: I just have to stay one lesson ahead of the kid.*

This is an admittedly low bar. It probably goes without saying, but you should really not fake it. Before teaching the basics to others, get some practice in yourself, and some basic sense of what the experience is like.

Then, share it.

References

Aurobindo, Sri. *The Synthesis of Yoga* (1948).

Austin MD, James H. *Zen and the Brain: Toward an Understanding of Meditation and Consciousness* (Boston: MIT 1998).

Austin MD, James H. *Meditating Selflessly: Practical Neural Zen* (Boston: MIT 2011).

Batchelor, Steven. *Buddhism Without Beliefs: A Contemporary Guide to Awakening* (New York: Riverhead Books, 1997).

Batchelor, Steven. *Verses from the Center: A Buddhist Vision of the Sublime* (New York: Riverhead Books, 2000).

Boorstein, Sylvia. *Don't Just Do Something, Sit There: A Mindfulness Retreat with Sylvia Boorstein* (New York: Harper One, 1996).

Boyle, Richard. *Realizing Awakened Consciousness: Interviews with Buddhist Teachers and a New Perspective on the Mind* (New York: Columbia University Press, 2015).

Dennett PhD, Daniel. *Content and Consciousness* (London: Routledge, 1969).

Gelernter, David. *The Tides of Mind: Uncovering the Spectrum of Consciousness* (New York: Norton, 2016).

Greene PhD, Brian. *The Elegant Universe: Superstrings, Hidden Dimensions, and the Quest for the Ultimate Theory* (New York: Norton, 2010).

Grof MD, Stanislav. *The Holotropic Mind: The Three Levels of Human Consciousness and How They Shape Our Lives* (New York: HarperCollins, 1993).

H.H. Dalai Lama. *Beyond Religion: Ethics for a Whole World* (New York: Houghton Mifflin, 2011).

Hanson PhD, Rick with Mendius MD, Richard. *Buddha's Brain: The Practical Neuroscience of Happiness, Love, and Wisdom* (Oakland, CA: New Harbinger Publications, 2009).

Harari, Yuval Noah. *Sapiens: A Brief History of Humankind* (New York: Random House, 2014).

Hatch MD, Steven. *Snowball in a Blizzard: A Physician's Notes on Uncertainty in Medicine* (New York: Basic Books, 2016).

Hawking PhD, Stephen. *A Brief History of Time* (New York: Bantam Books, 1998).

Kabat-Zinn PhD, Jon. *Full Catastrophe Living: Using the Wisdom of Your Body and Mind to Face Stress, Pain, and Illness* (New York: Random House, 1990).

Kabat-Zinn PhD, Jon. *Wherever You Go, There You Are: Mindfulness Meditation in Everyday Life* (New York: Hachette, 1994).

Karma Lingpa (translator). *The Tibetan Book of the Dead* (Boston: Shambhala, 2000).

Kumar, Manjit. *Quantum: Einstein, Bohr, and the Great Debate About the Nature of Reality* (London: Icon Books, 2008).

McLeod, Ken. *Wake Up to Your Life: Discovering the Buddhist Path of Attention* (San Francisco: Harper San Francisco, 2001).

McGilchrist MD, Iain. *The Master and His Emissary: The Divided Brain and the Making of the Western World* (New Haven: Yale University Press, 2009).

Nhất Hạnh (Thích.) *The Miracle of Mindfulness: An Introduction to the Practice of Meditation* (Boston: Beacon Press, 1975).

Pearce, Joseph Chilton. *Evolution's End: Claiming the Potential of Our Intelligence* (New York: Harper Collins, 1992).

Pearce, Joseph Chilton. *The Biology of Transcendence: A Blueprint of the Human Spirit* (Rochester, VT: Inner Traditions/Bear, 2002).

Pearce, Joseph Chilton. *The Heart-Mind Matrix: How the Heart Can Teach the Mind New Ways to Think* (Rochester, VT: Inner Traditions/Bear, 2012).

Pollan, Michael. *How to Change Your Mind: What the New Science of Psychedelics Teaches Us About Consciousness, Dying, Addiction, Depression, and Transcendence* (New York: Penguin, 2018).

Pribram MD, Karl. *Brain and Perception: Holonomy and Structure in Figural Processing* (Hillsdale, N. J.: Lawrence Erlbaum Associates, 1991).

Rovelli PhD, Carlo. *Seven Brief Lessons on Physics* (New York: Penguin, 2014).

Schroedinger, Erwin. *What is Life?* (Boston: Cambridge University Press, first edition 1944).

Siegel MD, Dan. *The Mindful Brain: Reflection and Attunement in the Cultivation of Well-Being* (New York: WW Norton & Company, 2007).

Singer, Michael A. *The Untethered Soul: The Journey Beyond Yourself* (Oakland, CA: New Harbinger Publications, 2007).

Vedantam, Shankar. *The Hidden Brain* (New York: Random House, 2010).

Wallace PhD, B. Alan. *The Attention Revolution: Unlocking the Power of the Focused Mind* (Boston: Wisdom Publications, 2006).

Wilber, Ken. *No Boundary: Eastern and Western Approaches to Personal Growth* (Boston: Shambala, 1979).

Wilber, Ken. *A Brief History of Everything* (Boston: Shambala, first ed. 1996).

Wilson, Edward O. *The Meaning of Human Existence* (New York: Liveright, 2014).

Acknowledgments

Sometime in the midst of a life of reading, many of us think that we have a book in us, that we have something useful or important to say. Sometime in that same life, most of us also think that no one really would give a rat's ass about that first idea. The delicate balance between the self-satisfying impulse and the rodent's gluteus usually tips rat-ward; less to do with the genuinely interesting things lots of us have to share, I suppose, than being scared off by the daunting task of knuckling down to the writing and braving the humbling process of putting it out there for judgment.

I can only speak to my own motivations. Aside from the aspiration of showing up on C-SPAN 2 at three in the morning somewhere down the road, my own "I should write a book" intention was driven by my gratitude toward the practice of meditation and a sense that it could be more accessible with some tweaks in understanding and teaching it. The whole malignancy-driven, "time may be short, time to nudge the cosmic football a yard or two ahead while I'm still here" thing kicked intention into action. While the every-so-often comment I'll receive on the order of, "aren't you glad you got cancer, since...?" elicits from me a grimace more often than a smile, I'll admit that putting these lessons to some good use has been as effective a driver as any in finishing *Practical Mindfulness*. Now that's it's complete, some words of gratitude are a joy to convey. I'm sure I'll leave some folks out; my apologies in advance.

Teaching Gratitude: One of the great blessings of my career at Stanford's Family Medicine Training Program has been the group of faculty professionals I've worked with, a clan with deep care in their hearts and skill in their clinical and educational work. The core of old farts that have been parked there since I arrived fresh out of residency—Drs. Bob Norman, George Kent, Dale Rai, Frances Sun, and Mike Henehan—truly personify the lovely Family Practice mission, which emphasizes prevention, healthy self-care, and respect for our patients' ability to learn and collaborate. I especially appreciate the commitment, goodwill, and tolerance for my occasional nonsense from my colleagues in our Behavioral Science Faculty, including Frances Respicio, LCSW, Kathy Mullins, MD, Mike Stevens, MD, and Robin Beresford, LMFT. Our late '90s (wow, we're old) brainstorming on how to apply mindfulness principles and tactics in our clinic was the root of much of what later developed into this book.

On the less science-y side of my meditative career, my love and appreciation go out to my retreat "family" at Clear Mountain Wisdom in Auburn, CA and my main teacher, Dan Jorgensen. A reluctant guru was Dan—he'd never call himself that. He's been a wise, gentle mentor and teacher; I couldn't have found a better person to guide me in this practice, in both my own development and confidence in bringing it to others. I miss him greatly.

After some work in teaching meditation in small groups of adults, developing a program to get the kids sitting was a natural extension. My appreciation goes out to my school partners at the Eureka Union School District, Assistant Superintendent Dave Del Gardo and teacher Jane Murnane, for their efforts in helping me launch the 123 Focus project—initially a classroom curriculum and now morphing into a podcast.

Publishing gratitude: The crack team at Mango has been spot on with modifications to shape the book to its aspirational ideal. My thanks to Chris McKenney, Hugo Villabona, Brenda Knight, Hannah Paulsen, graphic artiste Jermaine Lau, and especially my developmental editor, Yaddyra Peralta, who course-corrected some of my less-than-practical rhetorical flourishes with good sense and style. Editorial consultant Melissa Kirk has been my secret weapon, kind but firm in reining in some of my less attractive editorial impulses (which tend toward the ironically impractical, "look how smart these words make me sound!"); her experience in the business has been invaluable to me. Recognizing I needed some actual publishing chops, I offered *The Sacramento Bee* editorial page editor Dan Morain a (bloated, semicolon-laden) essay. To my good fortune, rather than hitting "delete," Dan unwittingly provided a brief but powerful consultation on precision and concision in the form, which I deeply appreciate. Thanks also to the late, great Ron Shoop, an East Bay publishing icon whom I met by happenstance—pinging off each other's snarky posts on Facebook. A brief and fruitful friendship followed, with Ron providing sage advice and referrals. Thanks also to my underpaid, well, unpaid focus group of readers/proofreaders/editors/"attaboy" providers. First is my good and capable friend Dina Burns, who provided a thorough first edit of the manuscript—how fortunate I am to have a pal who writes for a living! Dr. Lisa Goldstein, Liz Vigil, Ryan Sazima, and my patient bride, Dr. Tracy Brown Sazima, all weighed in on concepts, structures, and rewrites. Thank you to all for your helpful input and support.

Personal gratitude comes last. That starts with Mom's heart and Dad's discipline. My old friend Drew Ross, MD, has traded, bounced, and mix-mastered ideas and attitude with me for forty years since our first days at Johns Hopkins; he's shaped my worldview in so many ways. It's rare to have one of your closest friends also be a world-class radiologist for all of your complex MRI reading needs. (Everyone should have one!) I got mine—Joe Mersol, MD, a brilliant, funny, virtuous man. He's shouldered the miserable task of telling his old friend his cancer is back on a couple of occasions, which I wouldn't wish on anyone. Some remarkable doctors have helped save life and limb: Henry Grinvalsky, MD, Derrick Schmidt, MD, and especially Kern Guppy, MD, who has miraculously salvaged a wreck of a neck on three occasions. (Please don't retire.)

My own family has pulled me through this unusual decade. I have three amazing sons and a wonderful new daughter, all different in style but with a common bond of care and compassion. Ryan, Matt, Andy, and Arielle, thank you all for your love, patience and support. Thanks also to my wonderful in-laws Lois and Mike Brown, and my siblings-in law Griff, Scott, and Hannelore and the Brown clan. They accepted a quirky Midwesterner into their California clan. I miss Mike every damn day.

Lastly, to my love, my heart, my partner...you know.

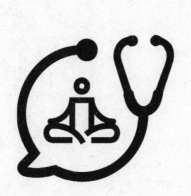

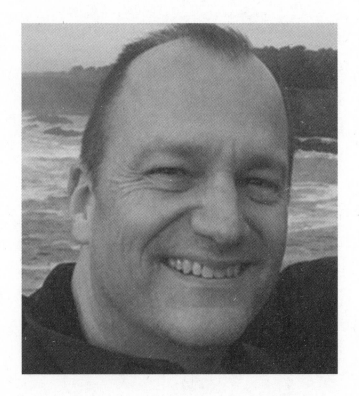

About the Author

Greg Sazima, MD is a board-certified psychiatrist practicing in the Sacramento area. He teaches physicians-in-training as Senior Behavioral Faculty at the Stanford/O'Connor Family Medicine Residency Program in San Jose. In addition to his clinical, teaching, and writing work, Dr. Sazima serves on the Boards of Directors of Snowline Hospice and Capital Public Radio.

Dr. Sazima was born and raised in Cleveland, Ohio. He graduated in 1983 from The Johns Hopkins University with a BA in Social Relations, earned his MD in 1987 from the University of Cincinnati College of Medicine, and completed his psychiatric residency training at the University of Connecticut and Stanford University Medical Centers. He started his private practice and teaching roles in San Jose in 1991. His current clinical, teaching, and writing activities include mindfulness practices, the MD/patient relationship, and physician wellness. His essays on mental health issues have appeared in newspapers and medical journals. *Practical Mindfulness: A Physician's No-Nonsense Guide to Meditation for Beginners* is his first book.

Dr. Sazima resides in Granite Bay with his wife, Tracy Brown Sazima, MD, a family physician in clinical and leadership roles at Kaiser Permanente, Folsom. The couple has three adult sons. Dr. Sazima has a deep interest in jazz piano yet only questionable skills in performance; besides piano, his other interests include hiking, cooking, kayaking, and, um, meditation.

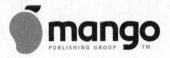

Mango Publishing, established in 2014, publishes an eclectic list of books by diverse authors—both new and established voices—on topics ranging from business, personal growth, women's empowerment, LGBTQ studies, health, and spirituality to history, popular culture, time management, decluttering, lifestyle, mental wellness, aging, and sustainable living. We were recently named 2019 *and* 2020's #1 fastest growing independent publisher by *Publishers Weekly*. Our success is driven by our main goal, which is to publish high quality books that will entertain readers as well as make a positive difference in their lives.

Our readers are our most important resource; we value your input, suggestions, and ideas. We'd love to hear from you—after all, we are publishing books for you!

Please stay in touch with us and follow us at:

Facebook: Mango Publishing

Twitter: @MangoPublishing

Instagram: @MangoPublishing

LinkedIn: Mango Publishing

Pinterest: Mango Publishing

Newsletter: mangopublishinggroup.com/newsletter

Join us on Mango's journey to reinvent publishing, one book at a time.